ONE STOP DOC

Renal and Urinary System and Electrolyte Balance

One Stop Doc

Titles in the series include:

Cardiovascular System – Jonathan Aron
Editorial Advisor – Jeremy Ward

Cell and Molecular Biology – Desikan Rangarajan and David Shaw
Editorial Advisor – Barbara Moreland

Endocrine and Reproductive Systems – Caroline Jewels and Alexandra Tillett
Editorial Advisor – Stuart Milligan

Gastrointestinal System – Miruna Canagaratnam
Editorial Advisor – Richard Naftalin

Musculoskeletal System – Wayne Lam, Bassel Zebian and Rishi Aggarwal
Editorial Advisor – Alistair Hunter

Nervous System – Elliott Smock
Editorial Advisor – Clive Coen

Nutrition and Metabolism – Miruna Canagaratnam and David Shaw
Editorial Advisors – Barbara Moreland and Richard Naftalin

Respiratory System – Jo Dartnell and Michelle Ramsay
Editorial Advisor – John Rees

ONE STOP DOC

Renal and Urinary System and Electrolyte Balance

Panos Stamoulos MBBS BSc(Hons)
Pre-Registration House Officer, Conquest Hospital, Hastings, East Sussex, UK

Spyridon Bakalis MBBS BSc(Hons)
Pre-Registration House Officer, William Harvey Hospital, Ashford, Kent, UK

Editorial Advisors
Alistair Hunter BSc(Hons) PhD
Senior Lecturer, Guy's, King's and St Thomas' School of Biomedical Sciences, King's College London, London, UK

Richard Naftalin MB ChB MSc PhD DSc
Professor of Epithelial Physiology, King's College, London and Guy's Campus Centre for Vascular Biology and Medicine, London, UK

Series Editor
Elliott Smock BSc(Hons)
Fifth year medical student, Guy's, King's and St Thomas' Medical School, London, UK

Contributing Author
Megan Morris BSc(Hons)
Fifth year medical student, Guy's, King's and St Thomas' Medical School, London, UK

Hodder Arnold
A MEMBER OF THE HODDER HEADLINE GROUP

First published in Great Britain in 2005 by
Hodder Education, a member of the Hodder Headline Group,
338 Euston Road, London NW1 3BH

http://www.hoddereducation.co.uk

Distributed in the United States of America by
Oxford University Press Inc.,
198 Madison Avenue, New York, NY10016
Oxford is a registered trademark of Oxford University Press

Whilst the advice and information in this book are believed to be true and
accurate at the date of going to press, neither the author[s] nor the publisher
can accept any legal responsibility or liability for any errors or omissions
that may be made. In particular, (but without limiting the generality of the
preceding disclaimer) every effort has been made to check drug dosages;
however it is still possible that errors have been missed. Furthermore,
dosage schedules are constantly being revised and new side-effects
recognized. For these reasons the reader is strongly urged to consult the
drug companies' printed instructions before administering any of the drugs
recommended in this book.

British Library Cataloguing in Publication Data
A catalogue record for this book is available from the British Library

Library of Congress Cataloging-in-Publication Data
A catalog record for this book is available from the Library of Congress

ISBN-10: 0 340 885076
ISBN-13: 978 0 340 88507 9

1 2 3 4 5 6 7 8 9 10

Commissioning Editor: Georgina Bentliff
Project Editor: Heather Smith
Production Controller: Jane Lawrence
Cover Design: Amina Dudhia
Illustrations: Cactus Design

Typeset in 10/12pt Adobe Garamond/Akzidenz GroteskBE by Servis Filmsetting Ltd, Manchester
Printed and bound in Spain

Hodder Headline's policy is to use papers that are natural, renewable and recyclable
Products and made from wood grown in sustainable forests. The logging and manufacturing processes are
expected to conform to the environmental regulations of the country of origin.

What do you think about this book? Or any other Hodder Arnold title?
Please visit our website at **www.hoddereducation.co.uk**

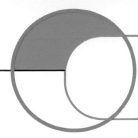

CONTENTS

PREFACE

From the Series Editor, Elliott Smock

Are you ready to face your looming exams? If you have done loads of work, then congratulations; we hope this opportunity to practise SAQs, EMQs, MCQs and Problem-based Questions on every part of the core curriculum will help you consolidate what you've learnt and improve your exam technique. If you don't feel ready, don't panic – the One Stop Doc series has all the answers you need to catch up and pass.

There are only a limited number of questions an examiner can throw at a beleaguered student and this text can turn that to your advantage. By getting straight into the heart of the core questions that come up year after year and by giving you the model answers you need, this book will arm you with the knowledge to succeed in your exams. Broken down into logical sections, you can learn all the important facts you need to pass without having to wade through tons of different textbooks when you simply don't have the time. All questions presented here are 'core'; those of the highest importance have been highlighted to allow even sharper focus if time for revision is running out. In addition, to allow you to organize your revision efficiently, questions have been grouped by topic, with answers supported by detailed integrated explanations.

On behalf of all the One Stop Doc authors I wish you the very best of luck in your exams and hope these books serve you well!

From the author, Panos Stamoulos

I decided to write this book after a colleague of mine invited me to participate in a series of books directed at medical students. I started writing it while I was still a medical student, after considering the current demands put on medical students by the current medical curriculum. I also used my experience as a medical tutee to tune it to a form that will be both appealing and easily absorbed for exam purposes. This book is not directed at replacing the standard textbook; its purpose is to challenge students academically and prepare them for their exams using an integrated approach towards all the key topics pertaining to the renal system.

Writing a book is a long and demanding process. It requires determination and perseverance to reach a form that will satisfy its goals, its author and its readers. I have watched it grow day by day and I am pleased to say that my work has been successful as well as fulfilling.

I thank Professor Naftalin and Dr Hunter for their invaluable input and advice during the birth of this book. I would also like to thank Elliott for trusting me with this work and his patience. I would like to dedicate this book to my parents and my godparents as a small token of appreciation for their support and sacrifice throughout my medical course

From the author, Spyridon Bakalis

'Whatever does not spring from a man's free choice, or is only the result of instruction and guidance, does not enter into his very being, but still remains alien to his true nature; he does not perform it with truly human energies, but merely with mechanical exactness'.

Karl Wilhelm Von Humboldt

I would like to thank the following people for the help, patience and advice: My family, Panos, Katerina, Zacharoula, Maria, Eleni and Petros, my co-author Panos and advisors Professor Richard Naftalin and Dr Alistair Hunter. Finally my friends who supported me throughout my medical years: George, Neil, Asim, Thanos, Vasanthan, Alex and Richard the house officers at WHH, and to all those I have no space for (I know who you are). Finally, to Heather who may have kept me out of trouble.

ABBREVIATIONS

ADP	adenosine diphosphate
ACE	angiotensin converting enzyme
ADH	anti-diuretic hormone
ANP	atrial natriuretic peptide
ATP	adenosine triphosphate
COPD	chronic obstructive pulmonary disorder
CT	collecting tubules
DCT	distal convoluted tubule
DNA	deoxyribonucleic acid
DT	distal tubule
ECF	extracellular fluid
ECG	electrocardiogram
ECV	effective circulating volume
ECV	extracellular volume;
ENaC	epithelial Na^+ conduction channels
GFR	glomerular filtration rate
ICF	intracellular fluid
ISF	interstitial fluid
JGA	juxtaglomerular apparatus
MAP	mean arterial pressure
$1,25[OH]_2D_3$	1,25-dihydroxyvitamin D_3
PAH	para-aminohippurate
PCT	proximal convoluted tubule
PTH	parathyroid hormone
RBF	renal blood flow
RNA	ribonucleic acid
RPF	renal plasma flow rate

SECTION 1

THE KIDNEYS

1. Label the following diagram showing the gross anatomy of the kidney. Each option can be used once, more than once or not at all

Options

1. Medulla
2. Cortex
3. Ureter
4. Renal pelvis
5. Adrenal gland
6. Pyramid
7. Major calyx
8. Minor calyx
9. Renal capsule
10. Renal hilum

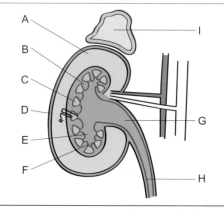

2. In the anatomy of the kidney

a. The inner part of the kidney is called the cortex
b. Nephrons are found in the medulla and cortex of the kidney
c. The pyramids are only found in the medulla
d. Collecting ducts are found in the pyramids only
e. Each kidney has four major calyces

3. Concerning the surface anatomy of the kidney

a. The subcostal plane is the surface marking used for locating the kidneys
b. The left kidney is higher than the right kidney
c. The inferior pole of the right kidney is about a fingerbreadth above the posterior iliac crest
d. The inferior pole of the right kidney is usually palpable
e. The hilum of the left kidney lies 10 cm from the median plane

EXPLANATION: THE ANATOMY OF THE KIDNEY (i)

The kidneys are paired, retroperitoneal organs that act as **filters** and control **H_2O**, **electrolyte** and **acid–base balance homeostasis**. They also have an important **endocrine** role.

Each kidney is made up from an outer **cortex** and inner **medulla**. The most important structural component of the kidney is the **nephron**. These are found in both the cortex and medulla; however, the **renal corpuscle** component of the nephron is only found in the cortex. The medulla contains the **collecting ducts**, which are concentrated in the **pyramids**. The pyramids are ordered so that their apical ends empty urine into the **minor calyces**, which in turn drain into a **major calyx**. There are three major calyces in each kidney. These drain into the **renal pelvis**, through the ureter, then down into the bladder.

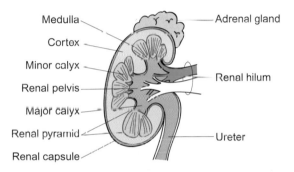

The **transpyloric plane** is the surface marking used to locate the kidneys. It is halfway between the suprasternal notch and the pubis at the level of **L1** and passes through **hilum** of the **left kidney** (which lies 5 cm from the median plane) and the superior pole of the right kidney. The **superior poles** of the left and right kidneys lie deep to the eleventh and twelfth ribs respectively (the right kidney is lower than the left kidney – it is pushed down by the liver which sits above it). The inferior pole of the right kidney is a fingerbreadth above the posterior iliac crest and is usually palpable except if the patient is obese.

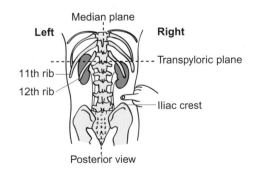

Answers
1. 1 – B, 2 – A, 3 – H, 4 – G, 5 – I, 6 – C, 7 – E, 8 – F, 9 – D, 10 – J
2. F T T T F
3. F F T T F

4. For each of the following choose the one correct answer:

Options

A. Diaphragm
B. Quadratus lumborum muscle
C. Pancreas
D. Second part of the duodenum
E. First part of the duodenum
F. Third part of the duodenum
G. Liver
H. Aorta
I. Inferior vena cava

1. Lies superior to the right kidney
2. Lies superior to the left kidney
3. Lies posterior to the right kidney
4. Lies posterior to the left kidney
5. Lies anterior to the right kidney
6. Lies anterior to the left kidney
7. Lies medial to the right kidney
8. Lies medial to the left kidney

5. The kidneys

a. Are 10 cm long by 5 cm wide and 2.5 cm deep
b. Lie between T10 and L3
c. Are retroperitoneal organs
d. Have superior poles that are both in the same transverse plane
e. Are positioned so their long axes are oblique

6. Concerning the kidney

a. The kidneys move about 5 cm during respiration
b. The collagenous capsule around the kidney readily expands
c. The kidneys are in direct contact with the eleventh and twelfth ribs
d. The perinephric fat helps holds the kidney in place
e. The renal fascia is the kidney's attachment to the diaphragm

EXPLANATION: THE ANATOMY OF THE KIDNEY (ii)

The relations to the kidneys are as follows: the **diaphragm** lies **superior** to **both kidneys**. The diaphragm, the quadratus lumborum, the psoas, the transversus abdominis, the twelfth rib and the three nerves (the subcostal, iliohypogastric and ilio-inguinal) lie posterior to the right kidney. The quadratus lumborum lies posterior to the left kidney. The **liver**, **second part** of the **duodenum** and the ascending colon lie **anterior** to the **right kidney**. The **stomach**, the **pancreas** and its vessels, the spleen, the jejunum and the descending colon lie **anterior** to the **left kidney**. The inferior vena cava lies medial to the right kidney and the aorta lies medial to the left kidney.

On entering the hilum the **renal vein** lies **anterior** to the **renal artery**, which is anterior to the renal pelvis. **Renal arteries arise** at **L1** to **L2**. The **right renal artery**, which is **longer**, passes posterior to the inferior vena cava. The renal artery splits to form an anterior and a posterior branch.

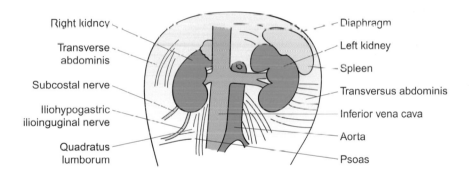

Each kidney is around 10 cm long, 5 cm wide and 2.5 cm deep, weighing about 150 g and lies between T12 and L3. Their long axes are oblique as the superior poles of the kidneys lie medially to the inferior poles.

The kidneys move only 3 cm on respiration; the movement comes from the superior-lying diaphragm. The surrounding **collagenous capsule** does not expand, therefore **inflammation** of the kidney may cause an **increase in pressure** within the kidney. The kidneys are separated from the eleventh and twelfth ribs by the diaphragm, though they are both related to both ribs. The perinephric fat surrounds the kidney, and lies outside the renal capsule, but inside the renal fascia. It provides protection from trauma. The tough renal fascia blends with the diaphragmatic fascia.

Answers

4. 1 – A, 2 – A, 3 – B, 4 – B, 5 – D, 6 – C, 7 – I, 8 – H
5. T F T F T
6. F F F T T

7. Label the diagram below of the renal microcirculation

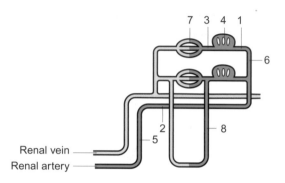

Renal vein
Renal artery

Options

A. Afferent arteriole
B. Glomerulus
C. Arcuate artery
D. Efferent arteriole
E. Interlobar artery
F. Vasa recta
G. Peritubular capillaries
H. Interlobular artery

8. Concerning the renal microcirculation

a. The glomerular capillaries have a different structure to other capillaries
b. The renal capillaries are all made of four cell layers
c. The renal vasculature contains three different capillary systems
d. The glomerular capillary system of the kidneys works at a higher intraluminal pressure than in any other organ system
e. To optimize glomerular filtration, the transluminal pressure in the glomerulus is always the same

EXPLANATION: THE RENAL MICROCIRCULATION (i)

The **renal artery** flows into the kidney and immediately branches into the interlobar arteries. They then run through the medulla, and sub-divide into the arcuate arteries, which then divide into **interlobular arteries**.

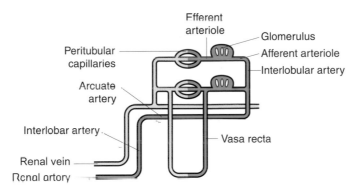

The **afferent arterioles** branch off the interlobular arteries and run into the cortex and form the **glomerulus**, the **efferent arteriole**, **peritubular capillaries** and **vasa recta**.

The **renal capillary system** in the kidneys is **different** and more complex from that in other organs. The differences are:

1. Capillaries are made from a single layer of endothelium, but in the kidney they are made of **four layers**: **endothelial cells** internally, sitting on a **basement membrane** (not cells), surrounded by special epithelial cells called **podocytes** (which have pores), which are in turn surrounded by a set of **Bowman's capsule cells**.

2. The renal capillary system consists of three sub-capillary systems: the **glomerulus**, the cortical **peritubular capillaries**, and the **vasa recta**.

3. The intraluminal pressure in the glomerulus is about **twice** as **high** as that in other capillaries, i.e. 50 mmHg. This can be varied and aids filtration.

9. Concerning the renal microcirculation

a. The glomerulus receives blood from the efferent arteriole
b. Twenty per cent of blood flowing into the glomerulus flows out through the efferent arterioles
c. The afferent arterioles from superficial nephrons run mainly in the medulla
d. The peritubular capillaries absorb and secrete substances from the kidney tubules
e. The efferent arterioles of superficial nephrons form the vasa recta

10. Concerning the renal microcirculation

a. The vasa recta lie in the cortex of the kidney
b. The vasa recta absorb substances from the loop of Henle
c. The descending wall of the vasa recta releases H_2O into the interstitium
d. The descending wall of the vasa recta releases Na^+ and Cl^- into the interstitium
e. The ascending wall of the vasa recta loses Na^+ and Cl^- into the interstitium

EXPLANATION: THE RENAL MICROCIRCULATION (ii)

Blood flows through the afferent arteriole, into the **glomerulus** and then out through the efferent arteriole. **Twenty per cent** of blood is **filtered** off by the glomerulus, whilst the remaining 80 per cent passes through to the efferent arteriole. The efferent arterioles (which have a smaller diameter than afferent arterioles) from different types of nephrons then form **two further capillary networks**.

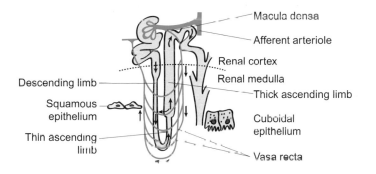

Efferent arterioles from **superficial nephrons** surround the tubular parts of the nephrons (hence the name peritubular capillaries) in the cortex, and are involved in nutrient transfer, removing reabsorbed H_2O and solutes and transporting substances to the tubules for secretion.

Efferent arterioles from **juxtamedullary nephrons** penetrate into the medulla, perform a U-turn and then run back up into the cortex. These arterioles form the **vasa recta**. Along their whole length the vasa recta are in close proximity to the **loop of Henle** and reabsorb substances from the loop (**countercurrent multiplier**). Permeability of the vasa recta to solutes in the loop of Henle varies: the descending **arterial** side **excretes H_2O** into the interstitium and **absorbs Na^+** and Cl^-, whilst the ascending **venous** loop **excretes Na^+** and Cl^- and **absorbs H_2O**.

The venous microcirculation of the kidneys mirrors that of the arterial.

Answers
9. F F F T F
10. F T T F T

11. **Label the diagram below of a nephron. Each option can be used once, more than once, or not at all**

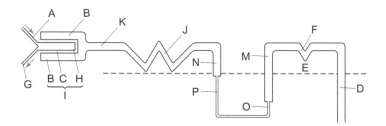

Options

1. Afferent arteriole
2. Bowman's capsule
3. Distal convoluted tubule
4. Bowman's space
5. Efferent arteriole
6. Cortex
7. Collecting duct
8. Glomerulus
9. Proximal convoluted tubule
10. Thick ascending loop of Henle
11. Medulla
12. Proximal straight tubule
13. Renal corpuscle
14. Thick ascending loop of Henle
15. Thin ascending loop of Henle
16. Thin descending loop of Henle

12. **Concerning the nephron**

a. Each kidney has about half a million nephrons
b. Sixty per cent of the nephrons are juxtamedullary
c. The renal corpuscle lies in the cortex
d. The distal convoluted tubules lie in the medulla
e. The juxtamedullary nephrons have shorter loops of Henle

EXPLANATION: THE NEPHRON

The functional unit of the kidney is the nephron, and there are around one million nephrons in each kidney. Each nephron can be sub-divided into two functional parts: the renal corpuscle (consisting of a glomerulus, a Bowman's capsule and a Bowman's space), which forms the ultrafiltrate, and the tubular system.

The **renal corpuscle**, the **proximal** and **distal convoluted tubules** are in the **cortex** of the kidney. The **collecting tubules** are in both the **cortex** and the **medulla**. In the latter part they run through the pyramids. The loop of Henle is also in both the cortex and medulla.

There are two types of nephrons: juxtamedullary (10–15 per cent) and superficial (85–90 per cent). Juxtamedullary nephrons have their larger corpuscles on the border of the cortex and medulla, and their longer loops of Henle penetrate deep into the medulla. Superficial nephrons have their corpuscles in the cortex, and their shorter loops of Henle barely, if at all, enter the medulla. The blood supply of the two also differs, with the efferent arteriole forming the vasa recta as well as the capillary network in juxtamedullary nephrons.

Answers

11. 1 – A, 2 – B, 3 – F, 4 – C, 5 – G, 6 – E, 7 – D, 8 – H, 9 – J, 10– M, 11 – I, 12 – K, 13 – L, 14– M, 15 – O, 16 – P
12. F F T F F

13. **Label the diagram below of the renal corpuscle. Each option can be used once, more than once or not at all**

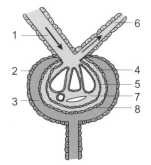

Options

A. Afferent arteriole
C. Capillary endothelial cells
E. Capillary basement membrane
G. Glomerulus

B. Bowman's capsule's cells
D. Bowman's space
F. Efferent arteriole
H. Podocytes

14. **Consider the renal corpuscle**

a. Blood flows into the glomerulus via the efferent arteriole
b. It is the site of nutrient transfer to the kidney
c. It is made up of a glomerulus and a Bowman's capsule
d. The glomerular capillaries contain small holes that allow proteins to filter through
e. The Bowman's capsule is made of a single layer of cuboidal cells

15. **Regarding the renal corpuscle**

a. The filtered material is dependent on size alone
b. The basement membrane has a positive charge
c. The filtration barrier is made up only of podocytes
d. There is high selective permeability of negatively charged ions
e. Myoglobin is filtered through the endothelium

EXPLANATION: THE RENAL CORPUSCLE (i)

The renal corpuscle **filters** the blood of **waste products**, forming an **ultrafiltrate**, the composition of which is adjusted by the tubular parts of the nephron to produce urine. The renal corpuscle has a glomerulus and a Bowman's capsule separated by a gap (Bowman's space).

The Bowman's capsule is made up of a single layer of squamous cells on a basement membrane.

The **glomerulus** is the **capillary network** that is fed by the afferent arteriole and drained by the efferent arteriole. The capillaries themselves are made up of endothelial cells, sitting on a basement membrane, surrounded by special mesothelium cells called **podocytes**. Some have a **negative charge** that influences substance flow through them. These cell layers have multiple **fenestrations** (small windows) that allow the blood to be filtered, with the filtrate passing into the Bowman's space and from there on through the nephron. The remainder of the unfiltered blood carries on through the efferent arteriole.

The **fenestrated endothelium** of the glomerular capillary wall acts as a **sieve** – H_2O and **small solutes** (urea, glucose, Na^+ and small proteins) may pass through. Negatively charged glycoproteins on some of the components of the filtration barrier permit the passage of neutral particles but restrict those with a negative charge. This explains the absence of albumin from the urine, but the presence of myoglobin.

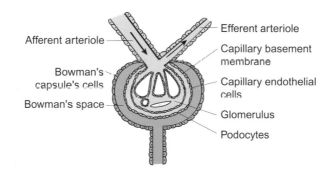

Afferent arteriole

Efferent arteriole

Capillary basement membrane

Bowman's capsule's cells

Capillary endothelial cells

Bowman's space

Glomerulus

Podocytes

Answers

16. **Match the arrows with the forces affecting ultrafiltration. Each option can be used once, more than once or not at all**

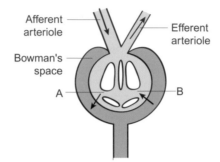

Options

1. Hydrostatic pressure in the glomerulus capillary
2. Hydrostatic pressure in Bowman's space
3. Effective hydrostatic pressure
4. Oncotic pressure in the glomerulus capillary
5. Oncotic pressure in Bowman's space
6. Effective oncotic pressure

17. **Concerning ultrafiltrate formation**

a. The oncotic pressure is dependent on proteins only
b. The oncotic pressure difference drives substances from the glomerulus into the Bowman's space
c. The efferent oncotic pressure is formed by the lower concentration of proteins in the ultrafiltrate than in the glomerulus
d. The glomerular oncotic pressure decreases along the afferent capillary
e. A balance between hydrostatic and oncotic pressure may be reached where filtration ceases (glomerular capillary oncotic pressure decreases along the length of the capillary)

EXPLANATION: THE RENAL CORPUSCLE (ii)

The ultrafiltrate is formed from water, salts and organic molecules – it contains the same salts and organic material as plasma and in the same concentrations. The driving force for ultrafiltration are the hydrostatic and oncotic pressures (the latter is protein dependent) within the renal corpuscle:

$$\text{GFR} = K_f \times [(P_{GC} - P_{BS}) - (\varphi_{GC} - \varphi_{BS})]$$

where GFR = **glomerular filtration rate** (mL/min), K_f = ultrafiltration coefficient, P_{GC} = hydrostatic pressure in the glomerulus capillary (50 mmHg), P_{BS} = hydrostatic pressure in Bowman's space (15 mmHg), φ_{GC} = oncotic pressure in the glomerulus capillary (25 mmHg), and φ_{BS} = oncotic pressure in Bowman's space (0 mmHg).

The **net driving force** between hydrostatic and oncotic pressures **favours ultrafiltration**. The overall **hydrostatic pressure** forces H_2O and solutes out into Bowman's space, but the lack of protein in the ultrafiltrate means the higher **oncotic pressure** in Bowman's capsule tends to draw it back again. As the ultrafiltrate is squeezed out, the plasma protein in the glomerular capillaries becomes more concentrated, thus the oncotic pressure in the glomerulus increases along its length. There is a point along the glomerulus where the oncotic pressure becomes so high that it equals the hydrostatic pressure. Beyond this point the forces are balanced and are said to be in **filtration equilibrium**, and no more filtration can take place.

Answers
16. 1 – A, 2 – B, 3 – A, 4 – B, 5 – A, 6 – B
17. T F T F T

18. Label the following simplified diagram of the ion transport system at the proximal convoluted tubule. Each option can be used once, more than once or not at all

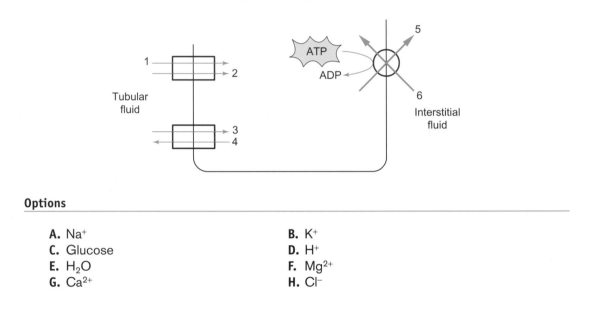

Options

A. Na⁺

C. Glucose

E. H₂O

G. Ca²⁺

B. K⁺

D. H⁺

F. Mg²⁺

H. Cl⁻

19. Cells lining the proximal convoluted tubule

a. Form a simple squamous epithelium

b. Have a large surface area in contact with the lumen

c. Reabsorb Na⁺ via the Na⁺ solute symport system

d. Are involved in secretion of organic acids

e. Have few mitochondria

20. The proximal convoluted tubule

a. Is the longest part of the nephron

b. Is the main site of solute reabsorption

c. Reabsorbs most of the water in the ultrafiltrate

d. Lies adjacent to the U-turn of the loop of Henle

e. Lies in the renal medulla

PCT, proximal convoluted tubule

EXPLANATION: THE PROXIMAL CONVOLUTED TUBULE (i)

From the Bowman's space, ultrafiltrate starts its journey through the nephron at the PCT, named 'convoluted' because it is so tortuous, and forms the longest part of the nephron. It lies near the glomerulus, and entirely within the renal cortex.

The primary function of the PCT is the reabsorption of the majority of ultrafiltrated solutes and water into the bloodstream. In a healthy kidney, almost 100% of filtered glucose and proteins (broken down to amino acids) are reabsorbed here, 80–90% of HCO_3^-, 67% of water, Na^+ and K^+, and 50% of Cl^- and urea. The second important function of the PCT is to secrete substances from the bloodstream. H^+ is secreted to help control blood pH, and is exchanged across the luminal membrane for Na^+. Organic acids and bases, including some drugs (eg. Penicillin) and their metabolites, are non-selectively secreted in the PCT to be eliminated from the body.

The cells lining the PCT are cuboidal and have a brush border of microvilli on their luminal surface. This gives them a large surface area for reabsorption and secretion. They are also rich in mitochondria that provide energy for active transport.

The effective reabsorption of almost all substances in the PCT relies primarily on the active transport of Na^+ via the Na^+/K^+ ATPase pump. For instance, glucose is reabsorbed with Na^+ from the tubular fluid via symporters that use the chemical gradient the pump creates.

Answers

18. 1 – D, 2 – A, 3 – A, 4 – C, 5 – A, 6 – B
19. F T T T F
20. T T T F F

21. For each of the following substances, match how they are managed in the proximal convoluted tubule

Options

A. Reabsorbed actively
B. Reabsorbed passively
C. Secreted actively
D. Secreted passively
E. Not dealt with in the PCT

1. H_2O
2. Na^+
3. K^+
4. Cl^-
5. Glucose

22. As plasma glucose concentration rises above normal, glucose

a. Reabsorption increases and then levels off
b. Clearance increases linearly
c. Is reabsorbed passively from the PCT
d. Is transported across cell membranes in the PCT in a similar way to amino acids
e. Is secreted by the Na^+/glucose ATPase pump

23. Regarding the PCT

a. It reabsorbs almost all the glucose in its first half
b. Glucose reabsorption is coupled to Na^+ reabsorption via the Na^+/K^+ ATPase pump
c. It actively absorbs proteins
d. It reabsorbs Cl^- passively
e. Urea is reabsorbed actively

EXPLANATION: THE PROXIMAL CONVOLUTED TUBULE (ii)

The concentration of Na^+ inside the PCT cells is low, and the interior is negatively charged with respect to the exterior, allowing Na^+ to diffuse passively from ultrafiltrate into the tubular cells. At the same time, the Na^+/K^+ ATPase pump actively expels Na^+ from the cells into the interstitial fluid, where it passively diffuses across to the vasa recta capillaries. This maintains the electrochemical gradient for further Na^+ entry, and also promotes the reabsorption of water by osmosis. As water leaves the ultrafiltrate, the concentration of solutes remaining increases. This creates a concentration gradient for K^+, Cl^-, $HCO3^-$, and urea to be reabsorbed by passive diffusion, whilst Na^+ entry creates a positive electrical difference that drives the reabsorption of negatively charged Cl^- and $HCO3^-$.

Glucose, amino acids, and other nutrients are reabsorbed by secondary active transport, using symporters. These rely on the Na^+/K^+ ATPase pump to keep the concentration of Na^+ low within the PCT cells. Thus glucose binds to a specific symporter with Na^+, and both are transported in the same direction, from the lumen into the PCT cell, driven by the Na^+ concentration gradient.

Please see page 48 for a diagram illustrating the PCT.

Answers

21. 1 – B, 2 – A, 3 – C, 4 – B, 5 – A
22. T F T T F
23. T F F T F

24. Concerning the loop of Henle

a. The ascending limb always contains thick and thin segments
b. The diameter of the lumen varies in the different segments
c. The loop of Henle begins and ends adjacent to its nephron's glomerulus
d. The thin segments have a cuboidal epithelium
e. The thick segments lie within the cortex only

25. Concerning the loop of Henle (continued)

a. Only 15–20 per cent of all loops of Henle are supplied by the vasa recta
b. The descending limb is highly permeable to water
c. The thin ascending limb is impermeable to water
d. The descending limb is highly permeable to Na^+
e. The thin ascending limb is impermeable to urea

26. The thick ascending loop of Henle

a. Is impermeable to water
b. Is freely permeable to urea
c. Passively reabsorbs Na^+ and Cl^-
d. Works to maintain osmotic pressures in the medullary interstitium
e. Contains cells that monitor Na^+ and Cl^- concentrations in the renal fluid

PCT, proximal convoluted tubule

EXPLANATION: THE LOOP OF HENLE

The **distal** part of the PCT becomes **straight** as it descends towards the renal **medulla**, and joins the first part of the loop of Henle, a **'U'-shaped** structure whose primary function is to determine the concentration of urine by controlling osmotic pressures in the medullary interstitium.

The loop of Henle can be divided into a **descending** limb, which lies entirely within the renal **medulla**, and an **ascending** limb, which returns through the renal medulla and into the renal cortex, ending beside the **glomerulus** and the afferent arteriole in a small segment called the **macula densa**. The macula densa of the ascending limb monitors Na^+ and Cl^- concentration in tubular fluid, to help in the regulation of blood pressure. About 15–20 per cent of nephrons have **long** loops of Henle that extend all the way through the renal medulla before returning back up to the cortex, whilst 80–85 per cent (cortical nephrons) have **short** loops of Henle that penetrate only the superficial region of the renal medulla before returning. The longer length of the **juxtamedullary** nephrons allows them to absorb water and solutes more effectively than the cortical nephrons. Only these nephrons are supplied by the **vasa recta**, which aids maintenance of osmotic pressure within the medullary interstitium, while both types have oxygen and nutrients supplied by peritubular capillaries.

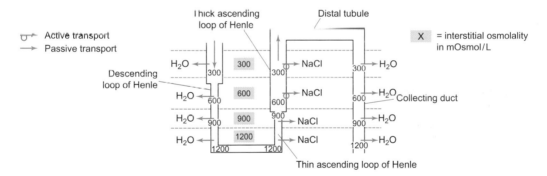

The descending limbs of both long and short loops of Henle are made up of **simple squamous epithelium** that gives the descending limbs a thin appearance. In long juxtamedullary nephrons this squamous epithelium extends some way up the ascending limb, before turning into cuboidal epithelium within the medulla, giving rise to the names 'thin' and 'thick' segments of the ascending limb. The short cortical nephrons have only a thick segment of cuboidal epithelium to their ascending limb. The lumen diameter is the same throughout the loop of Henle in all nephrons.

The descending limb is **highly permeable to water**, reabsorbing 15 per cent of all filtered water from the tubular fluid, but is relatively **impermeable to solutes**, including Na^+, Cl^- and urea. In contrast, the thin ascending limb is completely **impermeable to water**, but is **permeable to solutes** including Na^+ and urea. The thick ascending limb of the loop of Henle is **impermeable to water and urea**, and uses active transport to reabsorb solutes to maintain high osmotic pressures in the medullary interstitium.

Answers

24. F F T F F
25. T T T F F
26. T F F T T

27. Concerning the countercurrent multiplier system

    a. The cortical interstitium's osmolality is the same as that of the renal fluid flowing through it

    b. The countercurrent multiplier system plays a vital role in maintaining the osmolality of the cortical interstitium

    c. Renal fluid is at its most concentrated at the tip of the loop of Henle

    d. The volume of the renal fluid increases as it moves up the ascending limb of the loop of Henle

    e. Moving through the thick ascending limb of the loop of Henle the ultrafiltrate becomes hypotonic to plasma.

28. Below is a diagram of the solute transport pathways in the thick ascending limb of the loop of Henle. Match the letters to the numbered answers below. Answers may be used once, more than once, or not at all

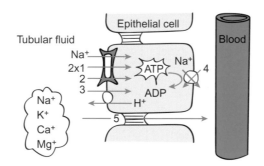

Options

    A. Na^+ **B.** K^+

    C. Cl^- **D.** H^+

    E. Transcellular pathway   **F.** Paracellular pathway

29. Furosemide

    a. Increases NaCl excretion in the urine

    b. Inhibits the Na^+/K^+ ATPase pump in the thick ascending limb of the loop of Henle

    c. Increases K^+ reabsorption in the thick ascending limb of the loop of Henle

    d. Reduces the volume of urine excreted

    e. Is used in the treatment of hypertension

PCT, proximal convoluted tubule

EXPLANATION: THE RENAL CONCENTRATION MECHANISM

The system used to create **osmotic gradients** in the **medullary interstitium** is known as the **countercurrent multiplier system**. This term derives both from the structure (two parallel limbs running in opposite directions) and function of the loop of Henle.

The system relies primarily on the ability of the **thick ascending limb** to actively transport Na^+ out of its cells through the Na^+/K^+ **ATPase** pump. As in the PCT, the reabsorption of all other solutes from the ascending limb is linked somehow to this function. These **solutes accumulate** in the **interstitial fluid** of the medulla and raise its **osmolality** above that of the cortex (which is isotonic to the renal fluid). The osmotic pressure in the medullary interstitium **increases** from 300 to 1200 mosmol/kg H_2O towards the tip of the medulla. Fluid entering the descending limb has the same osmolality as plasma, and therefore **loses** water down the water potential gradient into the medullary interstitium, **concentrating the renal fluid towards the tip** of the loop. **Countercurrent flow** of renal fluid within the descending and ascending limbs **magnifies or 'multiplies'** this osmotic gradient, and the **vasa recta remove** excess water and solutes added to the interstitium, to **maintain** the osmolality in a similar way.

Because the descending limb is relatively impermeable to solutes, salts and urea are not gained from the **hyperosmotic** medulla at this point. On turning into the ascending limb, **tubular fluid becomes increasingly hypotonic** throughout the ascending limb, as solutes are removed **without** any accompanying passage of water.

Fifty per cent of solute transport in the thick ascending limb occurs through transcellular pathways, and 50 per cent through paracellular pathways. Despite this distinction, **all** pathways, whether active or passive, are reliant on the Na^+/K^+ ATPase pump. This pump maintains a low concentration of Na^+ in the cells so that the movement of Na^+ out of the tubular fluid is favoured. This drives the $Na^+/K^+/2Cl^-$ **symporter**, and the Na^+/H^+ **antiporters** through **secondary active transport**. This solute movement in turn maintains a positively charged tubular fluid relative to blood, driving the reabsorption of cations including Na^+, K^+, and Ca^{2+} across transport proteins in the basolateral membrane (the paracellular pathway).

Furosemide selectively **inhibits** the $Na^+/K^+/2Cl^-$ symporter, **reducing** the amount of **NaCl** that is **reabsorbed**. As the reabsorption of water is driven by osmotic gradients, inhibition of solute transport therefore causes less water to be absorbed and a greater volume of water to be excreted. As a consequence, blood volume is reduced and this helps lower blood pressure. As a side effect, however, inhibition of Cl^- reabsorption also allows the charge within the tubular fluid to become less positive, reducing the drive for K^+ to be reabsorbed via the paracellular pathway. A patient treated with furosemide may therefore become hypokalaemic due to loss of extra K^+ in the urine.

Answers

27. T F T F T
28. 1 – C, 2 – B, 3 – A, 4 – B, 5 – F
29. T F F F T

30. Concerning the distal tubule (DT)

a. It is the longest part of the nephron
b. It lies exclusively within the cortex
c. Its cells have microvilli
d. It is mainly responsible for the regulation of Na^+ and K^+ excretion
e. It is permeable to urea

31. Concerning the DT

a. It does not play a role in acid–base balance
b. It has receptors for anti-diuretic hormone (ADH) and aldosterone
c. Aldosterone alters Na^+ permeability of the distal tubule wall
d. Aldosterone is synthesized by the adrenal medulla
e. ADH increases the distal tubules permeability to H_2O

32. For each of the following, use the correct term that describes how the distal convoluted tubule (DCT) deals with each substance. Each option can be used once, more than once or not at all

Options

A. Reabsorbed actively
B. Reabsorbed passively
C. Secreted actively
D. Secreted passively
E. Co-transported

1. H_2O
2. Na^+
3. HCO_3^-
4. K^+
5. H^+
6. Cl^-
7. Urea

ADH, anti-diuretic hormone; CA, carbonic anhydrase; DCT, distal convoluted tubule; DT, distal tubule

EXPLANATION: THE DISTAL CONVOLUTED TUBULE

The **DT** is the shortest part of the nephron, and lies within the cortex, close to the glomerulus. It is made up of the **DCT** and the **connecting tubule** (the connection between the DCT and the collecting duct).

The DT has **tall cuboidal epithelium** but with **sparse microvilli** and it is **impermeable** to both **H_2O and urea**. Its function is to **concentrate** the **ultrafiltrate** further, by absorbing up to 10 per cent of the filtered Na^+ and 15 per cent of the filtered H_2O. The DT also reabsorbs urea, and secretes H^+ and K^+.

Luminal Na^+ exchanges for intracellular H^+ across the luminal membrane via Na^+/H^+ exchange. The source of intracellular H^+ is carbonic acid whose synthesis is catalysed by carbonic anhydrase (CA).

The whole DT reabsorbs Na^+ by the same active method, via the $Na^+/K^+/2Cl^-$ symport. Na^+ enters the DT cells along its electrochemical gradient (the ultrafiltrate is more positive than the cells), along with one K^+ and two Cl^- ions. The Na^+ is then pumped out of the cell, into the peritubular fluid by the Na^+/K^+ ATPase active transport pump, with K^+ moving back into the ultrafiltrate via special K^+ channels. Cl^- passively follows Na^+ into the peritubular fluid. This system can absorb as much Na^+ from the ultrafiltrate as is necessary. The process of Na^+ reabsorption is influenced by the hormone **aldosterone**, which is released by the adrenal cortex.

ADH increases the permeability of the DT to H_2O altering the amount of H_2O reabsorbed producing hypertonic urine. The H_2O is withdrawn by osmosis into the interstitium.

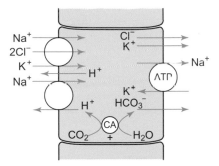

33. The juxtaglomerular apparatus (JGA)

a. Lies adjacent to the glomerulus
b. Contains granular cells which synthesize renin
c. Regulates the GFR
d. Is involved with the renin–angiotensin–aldosterone system
e. Is made up of two cell types

34. Concerning the JGA

a. Extraglomerular mesangial cells are an extension of the mesangium
b. Extraglomerular mesangial cells are closely packed columnar epithelial cells
c. Granular cells lie by the afferent arteriole only
d. The macula densa produces and releases rennin
e. The macula densa is a specialized zone associated with the thick ascending loop of Henle

35. Mesangial cells

a. Provide structural support for the glomerular capillaries
b. Regulate glomerular capillary flow rate
c. Have phagocytic functions
d. Are of three types
e. Do not synthesize erythropoietin

GFR, glomerular filtration rate; JGA, juxtaglomerular apparatus; RBF, renal blood flow

EXPLANATION: THE JUXTAGLOMERULAR APPARATUS AND THE MESANGIUM

The **JGA** is adjacent to the point where the thick ascending loop of Henle ascends to meet its corresponding glomerulus. The JGA has a role in **auto-regulation** of RBF and **GFR** and consists of **extraglomerular** (agranular cells) **cells** (effectively an extension of the mesangium), **macula densa cells** (a mass of closely packed cuboidal epithelial cells) and **granular cells**.

There are two types of **mesangial cells**: those that exist inside the glomerulus and those outside it (extraglomerular mesangial cells). The mesangial cells' function is to provide structural support to the glomerular capillaries, and by contraction they can alter the capillary surface area thus altering **capillary blood flow** and altering the **GFR**. The cells have **angiotensin II receptors** and myosin filaments that allow the cells to react to blood volume and concentration and to contract respectively. The other functions include phagocytosis, secretion of extracellular matrix and prostaglandins. **Erythropoietin**, which regulates erythropoietic activity, is also produced by the mesangium. Its production is controlled in a proportional manner by the O_2 tension in the kidneys.

The macula densa acts as a sensor that regulates juxtaglomerular function by monitoring Na^+ and Cl^- levels in the distal tubule lumen thus keeping the ultrafiltrate production at a constant level by altering the GFR. This is achieved via the renin–angiotensin–aldosterone system.

Renin is produced and released by highly specialized (granular) cells in the afferent and efferent arterioles.

Answers

33. T T T T F
34. T F F F T
35. T T T F F

36. Consider the collecting tubules (CTs)

a. They run through the cortex and medulla
b. They are closely related to the vasa recta
c. They merge to form ducts of Bellini
d. Cortical CTs contain cuboidal cells
e. Papillary CTs contain cuboidal cells

37. Regarding CTs

a. They consist of two types of cells
b. Dark cells have microvilli
c. Dark cells reabsorb Na^+ and H_2O
d. Clear cells secrete H^+
e. They are unimportant in acid–base balance

38. In the collecting tubules

a. H_2O is reabsorbed passively
b. ADH decreases permeability to H_2O
c. Urea is reabsorbed along with H_2O
d. There are specific Na^+ conductance channels in the wall
e. Aldosterone decreases the amount of Na^+ reabsorbed

ADH, anti-diuretic hormone; CT, collecting tubules, ENaC, epithelial Na^+ conduction channels

EXPLANATION: THE COLLECTING TUBULES

The **CTs** can be sub-divided into cortical, medullary and papillary parts and coalesce to form **collecting ducts**, which then combine to form ducts of Bellini, emptying into the **minor calyces**. The CT epithelium changes from cuboidal in the cortical collecting ducts to columnar in the papillary collecting ducts.

CTs are made up of two cell types: clear and dark (reflecting their appearance under light microscopy). Dark cells are organelle rich and have microvilli, whilst clear cells are cuboidal and organelle poor. Clear cells reabsorb Na^+ and H_2O, whilst dark cells secrete H^+ or HCO_3^-.

In essence, the CTs **permit passage** of the **ultrafiltrate** from the distal tubules to the minor calyces but they also have a role in **regulating acid–base balance** and altering the **final urine concentration**. This occurs because the collecting tubules run through the medullary interstitium, alongside the vasa recta and loop of Henle. The concentration of the medullary interstitium can cause passive H_2O reabsorption from the CTs. This is aided by **ADH**, which increases the permeability of the CT's wall and reuptake of water from the ultrafiltrate. The more ADH present, the more permeable the CT wall becomes, and the more concentrated the urine produced. Urea is reabsorbed along with H_2O in the distal collecting duct.

Apical epithelial Na^+ conduction channels (ENaC) allow Na^+ entry into the CT cells to be uncoupled from other ions or solutes, thus urine of different Na^+ concentrations can be formed. The amount of Na^+ reabsorbed depends on the amount flowing through the CT at any time. Na^+ reabsorption can be increased by the hormone aldosterone, which increases the number of channels in the apical membrane of the CT.

Answers
36. T T T T F
37. T T F F F
38. T F T T F

39. Renal clearance

    a. Is the measurement of the excretory function of the kidney
    b. Is based on Fick's principle of conservation of mass
    c. Is measured in volume per unit time
    d. Takes into account the volume of a substance that is returned into the circulation
    e. Is calculated by the equation $C_x = (U_x \times V) / P_x$

40. Concerning GFR

    a. The GFR is the volume of urine filtered by the glomerulus per unit time
    b. It is a measurement of the excretory function of the kidney
    c. The total GFR is normally around 60 mL/kidney/min
    d. A substance suited to measuring GFR must equilibrate fully between plasma and the glomerular filtrate
    e. A substance suited to measure GFR is neither absorbed nor secreted along the nephron

41. Concerning clinical measurements of GFR

    a. Inulin cannot be used to calculate GFR
    b. Inulin is reabsorbed by the proximal tubule
    c. Creatinine is a product of skeletal muscle metabolism
    d. Creatinine is freely filtered by the glomerulus
    e. Creatinine clearance is a satisfactory measure of GFR

GFR, glomerular filtration rate; RPF, renal plasma flow rate

EXPLANATION: RENAL CLEARANCE

Renal clearance is a measurement of the excretory function of the kidney and tells us the volume of plasma that has been 'cleared' of a substance that is excreted into the urine. It is based on Fick's principle of conservation of mass, that is, what flows into the kidney (via the renal artery), must flow out (either in the renal vein or the urine). Thus, for a substance X:

$$P^a_x \times RPF = (P^v_x \times RPF) + (U_x \times V)$$

where P^a_x = [X] in the renal artery (mg/mL); P^v_x = [X] in the renal vein (mg/mL);

U_x = [X] in the urine (mg/mL); RPF = renal plasma flow rate (ml/min); V = urine flow rate (mL/min). Rearranging this equation gives:

$$RPF = ((P^v_x \times RPF) + (U_x \times V)) / P^a_x$$

Assuming substance X is completely secreted and is not reabsorbed along the nephron (i.e. RPFv = 0), RPFa gives us clearance C_x, thus:

$$C_x = (U_x \times V) / P_x$$

Clearance has many uses, its main one being the calculation of **GFR**. GFR is the volume of plasma filtered by the glomerulus per unit time, assuming that substance X is used to measure it (GFR is normally 125 mL/min).

GFR is measured using either **creatinine** or inulin. The former is used in common clinical practice, and the latter in special circumstances (it is not endogenous and must be given intravenously). Creatinine is a product of **skeletal muscle metabolism**. It is produced at a fairly constant rate, and is proportional to body muscle mass. It is not perfect in its estimation of GFR because it is **excreted** to a small extent in the **proximal tubule**, but laboratory measurements of plasma creatinine overestimate its concentration by a similar amount.

42. Blood flow to the kidneys

a. Makes up as much as 10 per cent of cardiac output
b. Is controlled entirely by hormones
c. Decreases with sympathetic nerve stimulation
d. Is normally maintained within a narrow range by autoregulation
e. Is influenced by tubuloglomerular feedback

43. Hydrostatic pressure in renal glomerular capillaries

a. Falls by 5 per cent when mean arterial pressure falls by 5 per cent
b. Falls as the oncotic pressure rises along the length of the capillaries
c. Rises under the influence of angiotensin II
d. Falls as the afferent arterioles constrict
e. Is always maintained by autoregulation

44. When a patient's mean arterial pressure (MAP) falls by 60%

a. Vasoconstriction of renal arterioles will occur
b. Urinary output ceases
c. Glomerular filtration falls by about 60 per cent
d. Glomerular filtration remains unimpeded
e. Renal blood flow falls by less than 15 per cent

GFR, glomerular filtration rate; JGA, juxtaglomerular apparatus; MAP, mean arterial pressure, PAH, para-aminohippurate; PCT, proximal convoluted tubule; RBF, renal blood flow

EXPLANATION: RENAL BLOOD FLOW

Filtration of blood at the glomerulus is entirely dependent on the maintenance of **blood flow** and **blood pressure** through the kidneys, which makes up **25 per cent of cardiac output** (about 1.25 L/min in a healthy 70 kg man).

Glomerular filtration is promoted by the **hydrostatic pressure** within the glomerular capillaries. It is opposed by the **hydrostatic pressure** within the Bowman's capsule, and the **colloid osmotic pressure** within the blood (which is higher than in the tubules because of the presence of proteins).

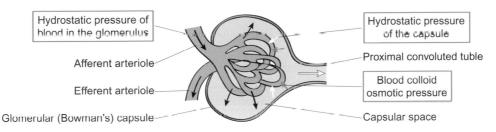

Hydrostatic pressure within the glomerular capillaries is determined by:

1. Renal arteriolar pressure at the glomerulus (positive effect).

2. Afferent arteriolar resistance (negative effect).

3. Efferent arteriolar resistance (positive effect).

If **mean arterial pressure** (MAP) falls, and hydrostatic pressure becomes as little as 40 mmHg, **glomerular filtration ceases**. This is because the opposing forces of Bowman's capsule hydrostatic pressure, and colloid osmotic pressure within the blood are now collectively as much as the capillary hydrostatic pressure.

A narrow range of renal blood flow (RBF) is achieved through a phenomenon called **autoregulation**, which works by altering arteriolar resistance to maintain hydrostatic pressure. It involves two mechanisms:

1. **Tubuloglomerular feedback:** $\uparrow$GFR $\rightarrow$ $\uparrow$NaCl delivery to macula densa $\rightarrow$ signal sent to $\uparrow$renal afferent arteriolar resistance.

2. **Myogenic mechanism:** relies on the intrinsic property of vascular smooth muscle to contract as it is stretched when arteriolar pressure increases.

Autoregulation only works at MAPs of 90–180 mmHg, when it is able to maintain a relatively constant RBF and GFR. However, RBF and GFR are also under humoral and neural regulation. Angiotensin II constricts afferent and efferent arterioles to reduce RBF and GFR. Atrial natriuretic peptide dilates the afferent arteriole but constricts the efferent one so that there is a small rise in hydrostatic pressure, to promote a raised GFR. **Sympathetic nerve activity**, triggered by dehydration or strong emotional stimuli/stress, will **vasoconstrict** the arterioles in a similar way to angiotensin II, thereby **reducing RBF** and **GFR**.

Answers
42. F F T T T
43. F F F T F
44. T T F F F

45. Consider loop diuretics

a. They are the second most powerful of all diuretics
b. Thiazide is one of the earliest loop diuretics
c. They appear to have a venodilator action
d. They are freely filtered into the glomerular filtrate
e. They can cause hyperkalaemia

46. Loop diuretics

a. Cause 50 per cent of the Na^+ in the glomerular filtrate to be excreted
b. May be administered intravenously
c. May cause hypovolaemia
d. Inhibit the Na^+/H^+ exchanger in the ascending limb of the loop of Henle
e. May cause metabolic alkalosis

47. Regarding loop diuretics

a. They inhibit the $Na^+/K^+/Cl^-$ symporter in the descending limb of the loop of Henle
b. They can cause hypercalcaemia
c. They can cause hypomagnesaemia
d. Frusemide is metabolized in the liver by glucuronidation
e. They are strongly bound to albumin

EXPLANATION: LOOP DIURETICS – RENAL ACTIONS AND SIDE EFFECTS

Loop diuretics are the most powerful of all diuretics, capable of causing 15–25 per cent of the Na^+ present in the tubular filtrate to be excreted; thus they are called 'high ceiling' diuretics. Main examples include frusemide (furosemide), bumetanide and piretanide.

These drugs act on the **thick ascending limb** of the loop of Henle and **inhibit** the transport of **Na^+** and **Cl^-** out of the tubule via the inhibition of the $Na^+/K^+/Cl^-$ symporter system. They also appear to have a venodilator action directly and/or indirectly through the release of a renal factor.

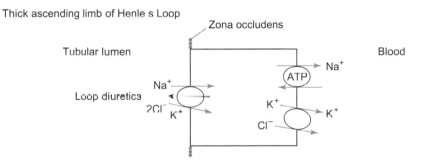

They are readily absorbed by the gut and can be given by injection (i.v.). They are strongly bound to plasma protein and so do not pass into the glomerular filtrate to any marked degree. They reach their site of action by being secreted in the PCT by the organic acid transport mechanism. The remaining fraction is metabolized in the liver (frusemide is glucuronidated).

Major clinical uses are in **chronic heart failure**, acute **pulmonary oedema** and **renal failure**. Major side effects include hypokalaemia, metabolic alkalosis, hypovolaemia and hypotension, hypocalcaemia and hypomagnesaemia.

Answers

45. F F T F F
46. F T T F T
47. F F T T T

48. Regarding thiazide diuretics

a. They act on the thick ascending limb of the loop of Henle
b. Metolazone is not a thiazide diuretic
c. They can cause hypokalaemia
d. They can cause hyperglycaemia
e. They can cause hypoglycaemia

49. Thiazide diuretics

a. Inhibit Na^+/Cl^- symporters in the luminal surface of intercalated cells of the distal convoluted tubule
b. Act as vasodilators
c. May cause hyperuricaemia
d. May be administered intravenously
e. Are tightly bound to albumin in plasma

50. Regarding thiazide diuretics

a. They can cause metabolic alkalosis
b. They can cause impotence
c. They can cause hypercholesterolaemia
d. They can cause hypercalcaemia
e. Diazoxide is not a thiazide diuretic

DCT, distal convoluted tubule

EXPLANATION: THIAZIDE DIURETICS – RENAL ACTIONS AND SIDE EFFECTS

Thiazide diuretics are the earliest true diuretics that were developed. They are not as powerful as loop diuretics. Examples include **bendrofluazide**, hydrochlothiazide, indopamide and metolazone.

They cause diuresis by inhibiting Na^+ reabsorption by the principal cells of the DCT. They achieve that by binding to the Cl^- site of the electroneutral Na^+/Cl^- co-transport system and inhibiting its action. They do not have any action on the thick ascending limb of the loop of Henle.

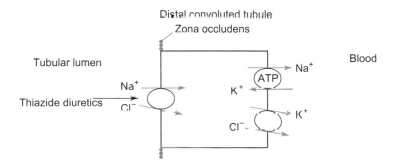

They have some extra-renal actions as well; they produce **vasodilation** and can cause **hyperglycaemia**. Diazoxide, a non-diuretic thiazide, has powerful vasodilator effects and also increases the blood sugar but its mechanism of action is a paradox; it opens membrane K^+ channels.

The thiazides are all effective orally and they are all excreted in the urine mainly by tubular secretion. Major clinical uses are in **mild heart failure**, **hypertension** and **nephrogenic diabetes insipidus**. Major side effects include metabolic alkalosis, hyperkalaemia and hyperuricaemia (with the possibility of gout) in the acute phase.

Answers

48. F F T T F
49. F T T F F
50. T T T T F

51. Spironolactone

    a. Is an ADH antagonist
    b. Acts on intercalated cells of the collecting duct
    c. Has a fast onset of action
    d. May cause gynaecomastia
    e. May cause hypolakaemia

52. Regarding triamterene and amiloride

    a. Amiloride acts on collecting duct principal cells
    b. Their action is via blockade of luminal Na^+ channels
    c. They can cause alkalinization of the urine
    d. Elimination of amiloride is mainly renal
    e. They are uricosuric

53. Osmotic diuretics

    a. Act on distal tubules and collecting ducts
    b. Are used in acutely raised intracranial pressure
    c. Reduce intraocular pressure by stimulating Na^+ loss by the kidney
    d. May cause hyponatraemia
    e. May cause hyperkalaemia

ADH, anti-diuretic hormone; DCT, distal convoluted tubule

EXPLANATION: K⁺-SPARING AND OSMOTIC DIURETICS – RENAL ACTIONS AND SIDE EFFECTS

Spironolactone, amiloride and triamterene are known as **K⁺-sparing diuretics**. They are used with K⁺-losing diuretics to prevent K⁺ loss and in Conn's syndrome. **Spironolactone** binds to intracellular **aldosterone receptors** in the principal cells of the **DCT** thus preventing the production of its mediator proteins. It is administered orally and its onset of action is very slow (several days). If used in isolation, it will cause **hyperkalaemia** and **metabolic acidosis**. Actions on steroid receptors in other tissues can cause gynaecomastia, menstrual disorders and testicular atrophy.

Triamterene and **amiloride** act on **collecting ducts** by blocking the luminal **Na⁺ channels** on the principal cell. Both are mildly uricosuric. They are administered orally and are well tolerated. Amiloride is excreted unchanged in the urine and triamterene is partly metabolized in the liver and partly excreted unchanged in the urine. Major side effects are **hyperkalaemia** and **metabolic acidosis**.

Osmotic diuretics (mannitol) are pharmacologically inert substances. They are **freely filtered** in the **glomerulus** but not reabsorbed by the nephron. Within the nephron, their main action is to passively draw **H₂O** into the lumen of the **proximal tubule, descending limb** of the loop of Henle and the **collecting tubules**. Their major uses are in **cerebral oedema** (acutely raised intracranial pressure), **glaucoma** (raised intraocular pressure) and prevention of **acute renal failure**. The first two effects do not have anything to do with the kidneys; instead they cause H₂O extraction from the brain and the eye. They are usually given intravenously. Major side effects are transient hypervolaemia and hyponatraemia and they are contraindicated in patients who are anuric.

Answers

51. F F F T F
52. T T T T T
53. F T F T T

54. Concerning glomerulonephritis

a. Glomerulonephritis is always due to immunological processes
b. All patients are symptomatic
c. Haematuria is a common symptom
d. Proteinuria is a common symptom
e. Glomerulonephritis never causes renal failure

55. Concerning the mechanisms of glomerulonephritis

a. Antigen–antibody complexes causing glomerulonephritis can only form within the glomerulus
b. Antigens are only bacterial
c. Parasites can act as antigens
d. Host DNA can act as an antigen
e. Drugs are not known to cause glomerulonephrtis

56. Concerning the mechanisms of glomerulonephritis

a. Immune complex glomerulonephritis accounts for 5 per cent of all cases of glomerulonephritis
b. Circulating antigen–antibody complexes that become trapped set off the complement cascade
c. There is no inflammation of the glomerulus
d. The basement membrane of the glomerulus is disrupted
e. *In situ* complex formation causes large amounts of glomerular inflammation

57. Anti-glomerular basement membrane antibody

a. Is an IgE autoantibody
b. Binds to an antigen on the podocytes
c. Is glomerulus specific
d. Does not cause damage via activation of the complement cascade
e. Causes 50 per cent of all cases of glomerulonephritis

DNA, deoxyribonucleic acid

EXPLANATION: GLOMERULONEPHRITIS

Glomerulonephritis is an **autoimmune** condition where the body's immune defences attack the kidney. Patients may present with haematuria, proteinuria, acute nephritis, chronic renal failure, nephrotic syndrome (proteinuria, hypoalbuminaemia and oedema) or may be asymptomatic.

Glomerulonephritis may occur as follows:

1. **Immune complexes**. In these cases **antigen–antibody** complexes become trapped in the **glomerulus**. The antigen can be **bacterial** (e.g. staphylococci or streptococci), **viral** (e.g. mumps or measles), **parasitic** (e.g. schistosoma), **drugs** (e.g. penicillamine), or the **host's deoxyribonucleic acid (DNA)** (e.g. in systemic lupus erythematosus). These complexes can either be circulating in the blood and become trapped, or be formed *in situ* (antigens that are trapped in the glomerulus are then attacked by antibodies). The damage to the glomerulus varies depending on where the complex is formed. This process accounts for **95 per cent** of all cases of glomerulonephritis.
- **Circulating antigen–antibody complexes**. The trapped complex sets off the immune response cascade that causes the glomerulus to become inflamed and damages the basement membrane causing haematuria and proteinuria.
- *In situ* **complex formation**. As the complex is formed within the glomerulus there is less immune response and hence no inflammation.

2. **Due to antiglomerular basement membrane antibody**. This **autoimmune IgG antibody** forms an immune complex with an antigen on the collagen of the glomerular basement membrane (it also attaches to collagen in the lungs). This complex sets off the **complement cascade** causing local inflammation and glomerular damage. This process accounts for 5 per cent of cases of glomerulonephritis.

58. Concerning acute tubular necrosis

a. There is necrosis of the renal tubular epithelium
b. It is most often caused by toxic substances
c. Toxic substance damage affects all tubule cells
d. Ischaemic damage affects all tubule cells
e. The process is irreversible

59. Concerning the stages of acute tubular necrosis

a. The oliguric phase is caused by dead tubular cells
b. During the oliguric phase the GFR is decreased
c. The altered GFR of the oliguric phase is not reversible
d. The polyuric phase is the result of dead tubular cell phagocytosis
e. During the recovery stage new tubular cells are formed

GFR, glomerular filtration rate

EXPLANATION: ACUTE TUBULAR NEPHROSIS

In these diseases the **tubular epithelial cells** and the **interstitium** are affected, resulting in poor renal function. There are two important diseases:

1. **Acute tubular necrosis**. In this disease there is necrosis of the renal tubular epithelium. It can be caused by **toxic substances** (affecting the proximal tubule) or more usually by **ischaemia** (affecting all tubule cells) of the kidney. The process is often reversible. There are three steps involved in acute tubular necrosis:
- The **oliguric phase** is the beginning of the disease where the dead tubular cells cause blockage, and hence an overall decrease in GFR resulting in less urine production.
- The **polyuric phase** follows when the dead cells are phagocytosed, thus unblocking the tubules, increasing the GFR and causing an increase in urine production.
- The **recovery stage** occurs when the newly forming tubular cells differentiate and begin to reabsorb substance from the urine, thus bringing renal function back to normal.

2. **Tubulo-interstitial nephritis**. There are many of these diseases, but the important ones are **interstitial nephritis** and **pyelonephritis**. Each of these can be re-subdivided into acute and chronic.

Answers
58. T F F T F
59. T T F T T

60. Acute renal failure

    a. Is defined by an increase in urine creatinine
    b. Is irreversible
    c. Develops slowly
    d. Can become chronic
    e. Can lead to death

61. The aetiology of acute renal failure

    a. Poor renal perfusion is the commonest cause of acute renal failure
    b. Sepsis may cause acute renal failure
    c. Renal vascular disorders never cause acute renal failure
    d. Glomerulonephritis can cause acute renal failure
    e. Urinary tract obstruction can cause acute renal failure

62. Concerning the symptoms and management of acute renal failure

    a. Oliguria is the commonest symptom
    b. Anaemia can be a presenting symptom
    c. Jaundice can be a presenting symptom
    d. Acute renal failure can cause electrocardiogram (ECG) changes
    e. Acute renal therapy is managed with fluid restriction

ECG, electrocardiogram; GFR, glomerular filtration rate

EXPLANATION: ACUTE RENAL FAILURE

Acute renal failure is defined by an increase in **serum creatinine** caused by a decrease in GFR. Acute renal failure develops quickly and lasts up to a few weeks, and can become chronic. Its aetiology can be put into three categories:

1. **Pre-renal**. This is caused by **poor renal perfusion** due to hypovolaemia (e.g. haemorrhage, diarrhoea, burns, sepsis, etc.) cardiac failure or renal artery obstruction, all of which decrease the GFR. This is the most common cause of acute renal failure.

2. **Renal**. This is caused by any disease that affects the GFR in any way (e.g. **glomerulonephritis, tubulo-interstitial diseases**) or internal vascular disorders of the kidneys.

3. **Post-renal**. This is caused by anything that causes **urinary tract obstruction,** for example tumours (including prostatic), kidney and ureteric calculi, ureteric strictures, etc.

Other than **oliguria** (urine production of less than 400 mL per day), patients with acute renal failure may be asymptomatic. Other signs and symptoms of acute renal failure include **pallor** due to anaemia, **hyperventilation** due to **acidosis, oedema** (both peripheral and pulmonary), **hyperkalaemia** (with or without ECG changes), **hyponatraemia, anorexia**, etc.

It is necessary to find the cause in all these patients, with a mixture of investigations (biochemistry, haematology, urine analysis radiological imaging and biopsy).

Acute renal failure is managed with fluid therapy to replace lost fluids. The serum K^+ level should be monitored closely as this can increase rapidly and lead to death.

Answers
60. F F F T T
61. T F F T T
62. T T F T F

63. Chronic renal failure

a. Develops quickly
b. Is characterized by a fall in GFR
c. Is reversible
d. Can last for years
e. Has the same causes as acute renal failure

64. Concerning the aetiology and presentation of chronic renal failure

a. Renal artery sclerosis is an important cause
b. Benign tumours are a known cause
c. Ureteric obstruction never causes chronic renal failure
d. Anaemia is a common presenting symptom
e. Urinary symptoms are always present

65. Concerning the management of chronic renal failure

a. Serum creatinine is used to monitor disease progression
b. The cause of chronic renal failure need not be treated
c. Diet modification is necessary as part of treatment
d. Dialysis is an early treatment method
e. All patients are suitable for transplantation

GFR, glomerular filtration rate

EXPLANATION: CHRONIC RENAL FAILURE

Chronic renal failure is also caused by a decrease in GFR, but develops more slowly, can last for years and, unlike acute renal failure, is not reversible.

Chronic renal failure has similar causes to acute renal failure, which can still be under the same three categories:

1. **Pre-renal**: due to renal artery sclerosis and hypertension.

2. **Renal**: caused by glomerulonephritis, malignant renal tumours, pyleonephritis, and polycystic kidney diseases.

3. **Post-renal**: evolving from chronic renal reflux nephropathy and ureter obstruction.

The patient's symptoms depend on the cause of the chronic renal failure, and include **polyuria, nocturia, lethargy, anaemia, clotting abnormalities, vomiting, anorexia, diarrhoea, confusion, coma, hypertension**, etc. Urinary symptoms are not always present.

Investigations are similar to those for acute renal failure, but extra tests such as crystallography are useful. Chronic renal failure is monitored by measurements of GFR and serum creatinine.

Chronic renal failure is managed by treating any causes of renal failure. Fluid therapy is necessary for either hyper- or hypovolaemia. Diet should be altered so as to control salt and protein intake. Blood pressure should be controlled as should hyperlipidaemia. **Dialysis** is necessary when the serum creatinine level rises (and therefore GFR has decreased) beyond a certain level (known as end-stage renal failure), or when symptoms seriously affect the patient's life. Transplantation may be an option in some patients.

Answers
63. F T F T F
64. T F F T F
65. T F T F F

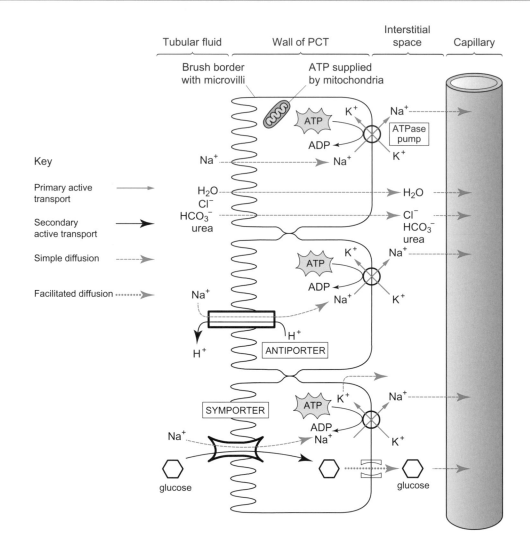

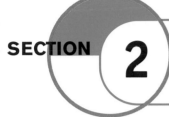

THE URINARY TRACT

THE URINARY TRACT

1. The ureters

a. Contain smooth muscle in their walls
b. Are non-expansile structures
c. Are made up of three layers of muscle along their whole length
d. Have an inner layer of circular muscle
e. Permit passage of urine under the action of gravity only

2. Consider the structure of the ureters

a. The lower third is the same histologically as the bladder
b. They have three layers of smooth muscle throughout
c. Longitudinal muscle is always deep to circular muscle
d. Ureters are expansile
e. Muscle layers are surrounded only by a layer of adventitia

3. Regarding the ureteric blood, lymphatic and nervous supply

a. The aorta is the ureters' only arterial supply
b. The inferior vena cava ultimately receives all ureteric venous blood
c. Lymph drainage of the ureters is partly to the lumbar lymph nodes
d. The ureters' nerve supply is autonomic
e. The ureters are supplied by spinal segments T11–L4

EXPLANATION: THE URETERS (i)

The **ureters** take urine from the **kidneys** to the **bladder**. They are formed from the **major calyces** that merge in the **renal pelvis**, and from here run down to the bladder. Ureteric walls are very similar to the wall of the bladder. They contain **urothelium**, which is a **specialized epithelium**. The ureters are made up of two layers of **smooth muscle** arranged as an inner longitudinal layer and an outer circular layer. The lower third of the ureter contains another outer longitudinal layer. The muscle provides the **peristaltic movement** of the ureters that propels boluses of urine along their length to the bladder.

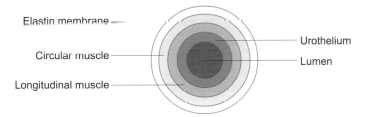

The ureters can be divided into **abdominal** and **pelvic** parts. Each has a different blood, lymphatic and nervous supply. The abdominal ureters receive their blood supply from the **gonadal arteries** (inferior section), **abdominal aorta** (middle section) and the **renal arteries** (superior section). Their venous drainage is via the **renal and gonadal veins**. The lymphatic vessels of the abdominal ureters drain to the common iliac lymph nodes and lumbar lymph nodes. The pelvic ureters receive their arterial supply from the closely associated **internal iliac artery** and the **inferior vesical artery** (males) or **uterine artery** (females). Venous drainage is via the **internal iliac vein**. Pelvic ureter lymph nodes drain into the lumbar, internal iliac, external iliac and common iliac lymph nodes.

The ureters' nerve supply is from the renal, aortic, superior and inferior hypogastric (autonomic) plexuses. These are associated with spinal ganglia at T11 to L2.

Answers
1. T F F F T
2. F F F T T
3. F T T T F

4. Concerning the anatomy of the ureters

a. They are 50 cm long (from kidney to bladder)
b. The ureters are only partially retroperitoneal
c. They are anatomically constricted in three places
d. Their constricted areas can be occluded by calculi
e. The ureters enter the bladder near its base

5. Answer the following questions with the options below. Each option can be used once, more than once or not at all

Options

A. Psoas major
B. Quadratus lumborum
C. Sacrospinalis
D. Tips of the transverse processes
E. The mid-clavicular line
F. Bifurcation of the common iliac arteries
G. Aortic bifurcation
H. Lateral wall of the pelvis
I. Posterior wall of the pelvis
J. Pubic crest
K. Internal iliac artery
L. External iliac artery
M. Levator ani
N. Obturator internus
O. Piriformis
P. Coccygeus

1. The abdominal part of each ureter runs along which muscle?
2. Which anatomical landmark is used to find the run of the ureter?
3. At which point do the ureters enter the pelvis?
4. Over which part of the pelvis do the ureters run?
5. Which artery is associated with the ureters within the pelvis?
6. Over which muscle does the ureter pass before entering the bladder?

EXPLANATION: THE URETERS (ii)

The ureters are 25–30 cm long, and half of this is in the abdomen (abdominal ureter) and the other half is in the pelvis (pelvic ureter). Like the kidneys they are **completely retroperitoneal**. As the ureters leave the kidney they run inferiorly along the **psoas muscle**. Superficially (and on X-rays of the abdomen) the **tips of the transverse processes** are used as a landmark for the course of the ureters. The ureters enter the lesser pelvis, running anteriorly over the **bifurcation of the common iliac arteries**. Once they have entered the pelvis, they continue their postero-inferior course along the lateral walls of the pelvis running anteriorly to the **internal iliac arteries**.

Finally they alter course in an antero-medial direction, staying superior to the levator ani muscles, and **enter the bladder obliquely at its base**. This obliquity forms the anatomical valves that prevent urinary reflux (see page 55). Along this course the ureters are **constricted in three places**: the junction of the ureters and renal pelvis, where the ureters cross the brim of the pelvic inlet and during their passage through the wall of the urinary bladder. These are important because they are the main areas where renal calculi (stones) can become impacted.

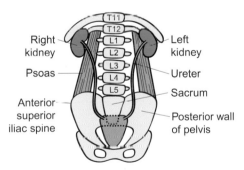

6. Concerning the bladder

a. Before micturition the bladder usually contains 500 mL of urine
b. In its relaxed state, the bladder is spherical
c. The wall of the bladder has the same structure as the lower third of the ureters
d. All three muscular layers are continuous with those of the ureters
e. The inside of the bladder wall is completely trabeculated to allow for expansion

7. Concerning the bladder

a. Urothelium is present as a stratified epithelial layer
b. Two anatomical valves prevent reflux of urine back into the ureters
c. Expansion of the bladder increases the chances of ureteric reflux
d. The internal sphincter lies inferior to the neck of the bladder
e. The bladder always remains in the pelvis

EXPLANATION: THE BLADDER

The **bladder** is used as a **store of urine** produced by the kidneys. Its existence allows us to only need to void urine 4–6 times a day, rather than have a constant dribble emerging. Before **micturition** it usually contains about 250 mL of urine though this can rise to at least 500 mL, which causes discomfort. The bladder is a **tetrahedron**, and is positioned so that the **apex is posterior to the symphysis pubis**, and its base anterior to the sacrum (the rectum lies between the two).

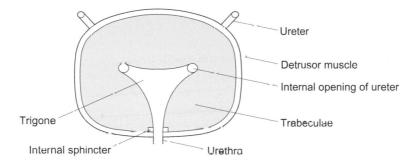

The bladder has the same histological structure as the lower third of the ureters. The **smooth muscle wall**, which is continuous with that of the ureters, has a special name in the bladder; it is called the **detrusor** muscle and is thrown into folds called **trabeculae**. The bladder also contains **elastic fibres**, which, combined with the trabeculated detrusor wall, provide the mechanism of contraction during micturition. The looseness of the layers of muscle gives the bladder its capability of expansion to accommodate large amounts of urine.

There are two systems that prevent **reflux** of urine from the bladder to the ureters during micturition. The first is due to the **oblique** way the ureters enter the bladder creating a functional valve (the **vesico-ureteric valve**). The second system only involves the musculature of the bladder. As the bladder distends, its musculature becomes increasingly non-flexible, and thus at the junction of the ureters with the bladder it becomes harder for urine to pass through this junction, hence stopping reflux during micturition.

Answers

6. F F T T F
7. T F F T F

8. Match the anatomical statement with the options below. Each option can be used once, more than once or not at all

Options

    A. In the male bladder
    B. In the female bladder
    C. In both sexes
    D. In neither sex

    1. The bladder is surrounded by visceral peritoneum
    2. The bladder lies posterior to the symphysis pubis
    3. The bladder has a lateral relation with the obturator internus
    4. The bladder has a lateral relation with the levator ani
    5. The bladder has a posterior relation to the rectum
    6. The bladder has a superior relation to the vesico-uterine pouch
    7. The bladder has a superior relation to the sigmoid colon
    8. The bladder is surrounded by parietal peritoneum

9. Concerning the bladder innervation

    a. The bladder is controlled by the autonomic nervous system
    b. Sympathetic nerve fibres arise from T11 to L2
    c. Sympathetic fibres are motor to the internal sphincter
    d. Parasympathetic fibres arise from S2 to S5
    e. Parasympathetic fibres are inhibitory to the detrusor muscle

10. Concerning the bladder vasculature

    a. The bladder vasculature differs between genders
    b. The internal iliac artery provides a blood supply directly
    c. In females the uterine artery exclusively supplies the bladder
    d. The vesicular venous plexus drains blood away from the bladder
    e. The external iliac lymph nodes are the prime site of lymph drainage

EXPLANATION: THE ANATOMY OF THE BLADDER

Anterior to the bladder is the symphysis pubis. Laterally in both sexes the bladder is related to the obturator internus and levator ani. Posteriorly, the association changes depending on the sex, in males it is the rectum, and in females the vagina. As with the posterior relation of the bladder, the superior relations are sex dependent. In the male the bladder is covered by the peritoneum and the sigmoid colon. In the female part of the bladder is covered by the uterus, and the rest, as with the male, by the sigmoid colon. The whole superior surface of the bladder is covered in parietal peritoneum.

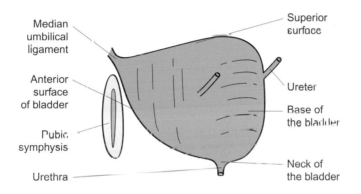

The urethra exits the bladder at the most inferior part of the bladder, which is called the neck. Just inferior to the neck there is a muscular sphincter, the internal sphincter. When this is closed the bladder collects urine and expands. When this sphincter relaxes, the urine is passed out via the urethra.

The superior and inferior vesicular branches of the internal iliac artery supply the bladder. In females the vaginal arteries supply some of the bladder, and in males the inferior vesicular arteries assist in blood supply. Venous drainage is via the vesicle venous plexus to the internal iliac vein. Lymph is drained along the vesicular blood vessels to the external iliac lymph nodes.

The bladder is controlled by the **autonomic nervous system**, and has both **sympathetic and parasympathetic** input. Sympathetic nerve fibres arise from T11 to L2, and innervate the bladder via the vesicular nerve plexus. They are **motor** to the **internal sphincter** and **inhibitory** to the **detrusor muscle**. Parasympathetic fibres arise form S2 to S4, (the pelvic splanchnic nerves). These are inhibitory to the internal sphincter and motor to the detrusor muscle. As the bladder distends it sends signals to the spinal cord through sensory fibres. Once it has reached a certain level of distension **parasympathetic** fibres on the bladder adventitia trigger **micturition**.

Answers

8. 1 – D, 2 – C, 3 – C, 4 – C, 5 – A, 6 – B, 7 – C, 8 – D
9. T T T F F
10. F F F T T

11. Concerning the urethra

Options

A. In males
B. In females
C. In both genders
D. In neither gender

1. It begins at the internal urethral meatus
2. It functions as part of the reproductive system
3. It is lined with stratified squamous epithelium only
4. It is under voluntary control
5. It has one external sphincter

12. Concerning the urethra

a. It is the same length in males and females
b. It is anatomically the same in males and females
c. It has the same functions in males in females
d. The urogenital diaphragm provides a voluntary sphincter muscle
e. The female urethra opens anterior to the clitoris

13. Concerning the male urethra

a. There are four parts to the male urethra
b. The nervous supply is autonomic
c. The penile urethra has stratified squamous epithelium
d. The penile urethra passes through the corpus cavernosum
e. The male urethra has only one arterial blood supply

EXPLANATION: THE URETHRA

The **urethra** is the tube that carries urine out from the bladder. See below for a diagram of the male urethra. The urethra is lined with **stratified squamous epithelium** in the meatal and parameatal parts. The muscular wall of the urethra is continuous with the smooth muscle of the bladder, and is under **involuntary control**. There is one **external voluntary sphincter** made up of the urogenital diaphragm muscles, that achieves voluntary urinary continence.

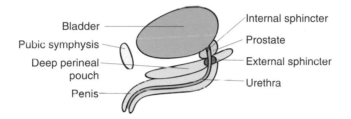

The female urethra is only 5 cm long and opens between the clitoris and the vagina. The male urethra is 20–25 cm long and opens at the external urethral meatus. There are **three identifiable parts** in the male urethra.

1. The **prostatic urethra** is the most proximal part. It runs through the prostate, where the ejaculatory ducts empty their contents into the urethra, and ends at the external sphincter.

2. The **membranous urethra** is the shortest part and runs from the prostate through the urogenital diaphragm muscles, which create the external sphincter.

3. The final part is the **penile** or **spongy urethra**, which runs the length of the penis to the meatus. It is surrounded by the corpus spongiosum.

The first two parts are supplied by the prostatic branches of the inferior vesical and middle rectal arteries. The internal pudendal artery supplies the penile urethra. The prostatic and membranous urethra's venous drainage is via the prostatic branches of the inferior vesical and middle rectal veins. The internal pudendal vein drains the penile urethra. The lymphatic drainage of the male urethra is divided in three ways; the posterior (proximal) and membranous parts drain mostly to the internal iliac nodes, the anterior (distal) part drains to deep inguinal nodes. In females, the drainage is to external and internal iliac nodes.

Answers
11. 1 – C, 2 – A, 3 – B, 4 – D, 5 – C
12. F F F T F
13. F T F F F

14. Regarding micturition

a. It involves a reflex arc through the lumbar spinal cord
b. It requires an intact extrinsic parasympathetic innervation
c. Distension of the urinary bladder is the trigger for micturition
d. Contraction of the urinary bladder can be voluntarily inhibited
e. The urinary bladder has no autonomic nerve plexus in its wall

15. The diagram below illustrates the neural control of micturition. Match the letters with the options below (+ denotes excitation, − denotes inhibition). Each option can be used once, more than once or not at all.

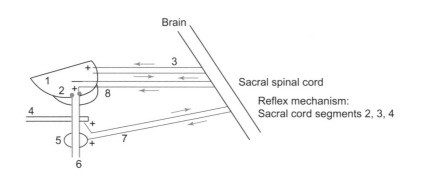

Options

A. Sympathetic nervous system
B. Pelvic splachnic nerves
C. Pudendal nerves
D. Detrusor muscle
E. Internal urethral sphincter
F. External urethral sphincter
G. Sphincter vaginae et urethra
H. Urethra

EXPLANATION: NEURAL CONTROL OF MICTURITION

Micturition depends on sensory information resulting from **distension** of the **urinary bladder**. Its innervation is dual: the **parasympathetic** nervous system detects distension and causes contraction of the **detrusor muscle**, whereas the **sympathetic** nervous system causes its relaxation (via beta-adrenergic receptors). The latter also innervates the internal smooth muscle sphincter and causes it to contract (via alpha-adrenergic receptors) thus closing the urethra.

The **reflex arc** controlling **micturition** is located in the **sacral spinal cord** and can be suppressed or enhanced by descending input from the **cerebrum**. The integrity of the spinal cord above the sacral level is essential for voluntary control. All relevant axons of the peripheral nervous system pass through the **cauda equina** and the mechanism of micturition can therefore be compromised by lumbar intervertebral disc lesions.

The urinary bladder fills until **a pressure of ~12 cm H_2O** is reached at which point the individual has the desire to micturate. If circumstances are appropriate the **skeletomotor** neurons innervating the external urethral sphincter, and possibly in the female the sphincter urethrae et vaginae, are inhibited and these muscles are therefore relaxed. The **sympathetic motor** neurons supplying the **detrusor** muscle and the **internal sphincter** are inhibited and these muscles are disinhibited and relaxed respectively. Finally, the pelvic **parasympathetic** neurons are excited causing contraction of the **detrusor** muscle. Overall, urine starts flowing through the urethra. Urine in the urethra sends signals back to the spinal cord thus enhancing the reflex.

Ascending signals make us aware that the critical pressure has been reached. Descending signals can be used to delay voiding by reversing the above effects on motor neurons, both skeletomotor and autonomic.

Answers

14. F T T T T
15. 1 – D, 2 – E, 3 – B, 4 – G, 5 – F, 6 – H, 7 – C, 8 – A

16. Regarding drugs and the urinary system

    a. Oxybutynin causes constipation
    b. Oxybutynin is an inhibitor of cholinesterase
    c. Prazosin can cause hypotension
    d. Prazosin is a selective $beta_1$-blocker
    e. Amitriptyline is used in nocturnal enuresis

17. Regarding drugs and the urinary system

    a. Oxybutynin is used in stress incontinence
    b. Terazosin is a non-selective alpha-blocker
    c. Lignocaine is used for urethral pain
    d. Desmopressin is used in benign prostatic hyperplasia
    e. NH_4Cl causes acidification of urine

18. Regarding drugs and the urinary system

    a. Oxybutynin can cause blurred vision
    b. Prazosin can cause dry mouth
    c. Distigmine is used for urinary incontinence in myasthenia gravis
    d. Oxybutynin is not used in patients with glaucoma
    e. Prazosin can cause severe hypotension

EXPLANATION: DRUGS AND MICTURITION – ACTIONS AND SIDE EFFECTS

Oxybutynin is a non-selective **muscarinic** receptor antagonist. It is used for urinary urge **incontinence**. It has many **side effects** including dry mouth, constipation, blurred vision, palpitations and heat intolerance. It should **not** be **used** in patients with severe **ulcerative colitis, gastrointestinal obstruction** and **glaucoma**.

Prazosin is an alpha$_1$-selective **adenoreceptor** blocker. It is used for **non-acute** urinary **retention**. It is employed in the treatment of benign **prostatic hyperplasia. Side effects** include hypotension, dry mouth, rhihitis, blurred vision and palpitations. Terazosin is also another alpha$_1$-selective adenoreceptor blocker.

Desmopressin is a **vasopressin** analogue and is reserved for non-resolving **nocturnal enuresis. Fluid overload** is the major **side effect** that can be produced. Amitriptyline, a tricyclic antidepressant, can also be used for this purpose but behavioural disturbances are common and toxicity can be a problem, so it is only used in very severe cases.

Distigmine is a **parasympathomimetic** drug. It inhibits the breakdown of acetylcholine. It is used for urinary **retention** associated with myasthenia gravis and neurogenic bladder (like in multiple sclerosis). Its side effects include muscle twitching, polyuria, nausea, vomiting, blurred vision, intestinal colic and bradycardia. It is **contra-indicated** in intestinal or urinary obstruction.

Lignocaine (gel form) is used to relieve the discomfort of **catheterization.**

NH_4Cl is used for urine acidification in recurrent **urinary tract infections. Side effects** include vomiting, **hypokalaemia** and metabolic acidosis.

Answers
16. T F T F T
17. F F T F T
18. T T F T T

ELECTROLYTES

1. Regarding the volumes of body fluid compartments

a. A 70-kg man has 42 L of water in his body
b. Intracellular fluid (ICF) accounts for 20 per cent of total body weight
c. A 70-kg man has 7 L of interstitial fluid in his body
d. Extracellular fluid (ECF) accounts for 40 per cent of total body weight
e. Plasma volume accounts for one-quarter of the ECF volume

2. Regarding the composition of body fluid compartments

a. Na^+ and its associated anions are the major ions of the ECF
b. K^+ is the predominant intracellular cation
c. Hypernatraemia describes plasma Na^+ concentration which is greater than 145 mM
d. The maintenance of Na^+ and K^+ concentration is achieved via the action of the Na^+/K^+ ATPase
e. The major extracellular anions are PO_4^{3-} ions

3. Regarding fluid exchange between body compartments

a. Water movement across a capillary is determined by the osmotic pressure differences generated by the different protein concentrations across the capillary
b. Hydrostatic pressure is an important determinant of cell membrane fluid exchange
c. Infusion of 2 L of normal saline (i.e. 140 mM NaCl) will increase the volume of the ECF compartment by 1.2 L
d. Infusion of 2 L of hypertonic saline (290 mM NaCl) will increase the ECF compartment volume by more than 2 L
f. The ICF and ECF compartments have the same osmolality

ECF, extracellular fluid; ICF, intracellular fluid; ISF, interstitial fluid

EXPLANATION: COMPOSITION AND VOLUMES OF BODY FLUID COMPARTMENTS

Total body **water** accounts for **60 per cent** of the body weight and is contained within two major compartments. The **ECF** compartment represents water outside of cells and accounts for 20 per cent of the body weight. The **ICF** compartment represents the water within cells and accounts for 40 per cent of body weight.

The **ECF** is subdivided into several compartments. The largest is the **interstitial fluid** (ISF), which is fluid surrounding the cells in the various tissues of the body (includes lymph, bone) and accounts for 75 per cent of the ECF. The remaining 25 per cent of ECF is **plasma** localized within the circulatory system. So in a **70-kg** person: total body water = 42 L, ECF = 14 L, ICF = 28 L, ISF = 10.5 L and plasma volume = 3.5 L.

Na^+ and its associated anions (Cl^- and HCO_3^-) are the major ions of the **ECF** and are the major determinants of the osmolality of the ECF. **Osmolality** is the number of osmoles per kg of solvent; to estimate plasma **osmolality** we use the following formula: $2 \times ([Na^+] + [K^+]) + [urea] + [glucose]$ ($\times 2$ because anions are associated with Na^+ and K^+). So, normal osmolality range is 280–300 mosmol/kg, Na^+ = 135–145 mM, K^+ = 3.5–5.0 mM, urea = 2.5–6.7 mM, glucose (fasting) = 3.5–5.5 mM.

Fluid exchange between body compartments can be separated in **capillary** exchange and **cell membrane** fluid exchange. The former is determined by the **hydrostatic pressure** and the **osmotic pressure** across the capillary in the following equation:

$$\text{Fluid movement} = K_f [(P_c + \Phi_i) - (P_i + \Phi_c)]$$

where K_f = capillary filtration coefficient, P = hydrostatic pressure, Φ = oncotic pressure, c = capillary, and i = interstitial fluid.

Fluid exchange across cell membranes is dependent on **osmotic pressure** differences; a change of osmolality in either ECF or ICF will rapidly lead to osmotic equilibrium by rapid water flow across the cell membrane.

Answers

1. T F F F T
2. T T T T F
3. T T F T T

4. Regarding water balance

a. Faeces are an important route of water loss from the body
b. The kidneys are responsible for minimizing insensible water losses.
c. In heavy exercise, water loss through the lungs is greater than water loss through the skin
d. The kidneys control water excretion by controlling Na^+ reabsorption only
e. An abnormal Na^+ concentration can be due to a water balance disturbance

5. Anti-diuretic hormone (ADH)

a. Is a polypeptide which binds to the collecting duct
b. Is released by the anterior pituitary
c. Its release is increased by a falling plasma osmolality
d. Is released by osmoreceptors in the hypothalamus
e. Is increased when there is an increase in blood pressure

6. Regarding ADH

a. It is reduced by a decrease in blood volume
b. It stimulates absorption of water by Henle's loop
c. It causes thirst
d. Its release is more sensitive to osmolality than blood volume changes
e. It increases the permeability of the inner medullary collecting duct to urea

ADH, anti-diuretic hormone; ECF, extracellular fluid

EXPLANATION: KIDNEYS AND ANTI-DIURETIC HORMONE

The **kidneys** are the major organs responsible for regulating **water balance**. Other routes include evaporation from the skin and the respiratory passages (insensible losses), sweating and the gastrointestinal tract. **Water loss** is regulated in the kidneys and it aims to maintain the osmolality of the body fluids constant. Because the major determinant of osmolality is Na^+ (and its anions), disorders of water balance will alter the plasma $[Na^+]$. Changes in **Na^+** balance alter the volume of the ECF and not its osmolality. The kidneys can control water excretion independently of other substances (e.g. Na^+, K^+), an ability that is essential for survival.

ADH or vasopressin acts on the kidneys to regulate the excretion of water. It is a small peptide (nine amino acids), which is synthesized in cells of the **hypothalamus** and released from axon terminals in the posterior lobe of the pituitary gland. Its secretion is mainly regulated by the osmolality of the plasma but both blood volume and pressure also have an influence. **Osmoreceptors** in the hypothalamus sense changes in the osmolality and they stimulate the cells that store ADH to release it into the circulation. **Volume** and **pressure** changes are transmitted to the brainstem via the vagus and glossopharyngeal nerves and then to the hypothalamus.

ADH increases the permeability of the **collecting duct** to water. It also stimulates the active reabsorption of NaCl by the **thick ascending limb** of Henle's loop and by the **collecting duct**. Finally, it increases the permeability to urea of the inner medullary collecting duct.

Answers

4. F F T F T
5. T F F F F
6. F F F T T

7. Regarding Henle's loop

a. Tubular fluid entering it is hyperosmotic with respect to plasma
b. The thin descending limb is highly permeable to H_2O
c. The tubular fluid is iso-osmotic with the interstitial fluid at the end of the loop
d. The thick ascending limb is permeable to H_2O and urea
e. The medullary collecting duct actively reabsorbs NaCl

8. Regarding Henle's loop in diuresis

a. The thick ascending limb passively reabsorbs NaCl
b. Tubular fluid at the end of the thick ascending limb is hyperosmotic with respect to plasma
c. The thin ascending limb is permeable to urea
d. The thin descending limb is highly permeable to urea
e. High blood flow through the vasa recta increases the reabsorption of NaCl from the thick ascending limb

9. Regarding urea and the nephron interstitium

a. Its concentration is highest in the medullary interstitial fluid
b. It is actively transported into it by the ascending limb of Henle's loop
c. ADH increases its reabsorption by the collecting duct
d. It is not essential for the generation of a hyperosmotic medullary interstitium
e. Low protein diets promote production of hyperosmotic urine with respect to plasma

ADH, anti-diuretic hormone

EXPLANATION: HENLE'S LOOP AND URINE DILUTION

The range of urine **osmolality** is from 50 mosmol/kg to 1200 mosmol/kg H_2O. The corresponding urine volume is 20 L/day to 0.5 L/day respectively. In order for the kidneys to excrete water maximally (i.e. dilute urine), separation of solutes and water must occur. This occurs in **Henle's loop**.

The following diagram shows the mechanisms involved in generating a **dilute urine**:

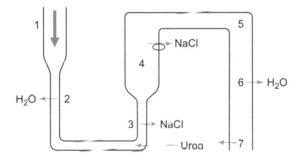

1. Fluid iso-osmotic to plasma enters Henle's loop

2. The thin descending limb passively reabsorbs water thus concentrating tubular fluid

3. The thin ascending limb passively reabsorbs NaCl thus diluting tubular fluid

4. The thick ascending limb actively reabsorbs NaCl thus diluting tubular fluid

5. The distal tubule and cortical collecting duct actively reabsorb NaCl and are impermeable to urea

6. The medullary collecting duct actively reabsorbs NaCl

7. Together all these events result in the production of copious amounts of dilute urine

Answers
7. F T T F T
8. F F F F F
9. T F T F F

10. Match the options below with the diagram letters. Each option can be used once, more than once or not at all (TDL = thin descending limb, TAL = thin ascending limb, MTALH = medullary thick ascending loop of Henle, DCT = distal convoluted tubule, CD = collecting duct)

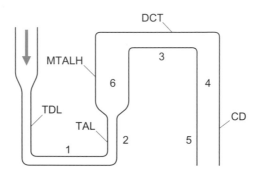

Options

A. Passive reabsorption of urea

B. Active reabsorption of NaCl

C. Passive reabsorption of H_2O

D. Active reabsorption of urea

E. Active reabsorption of H_2O

F. Secretion of urea into tubular fluid

G. Passive reabsorption of NaCl

H. Hypertonic Na^+ reabsorption

ADH, anti-diuretic hormone

EXPLANATION: HENLE'S LOOP AND URINE CONCENTRATION

Generating **concentrated** urine is essential in periods of sparse H_2O. The kidneys are really successful in generating highly concentrated urine. Again, like for dilution, the **medullary thick ascending limb of Henle's loop** is the key. This portion is impermeable to H_2O and urea. It actively reabsorbs **NaCl** and thereby dilutes the tubular fluid. However, it has to be noted that the reabsorbed **NaCl** accumulates in the medullary interstitium. This accumulation, together with that of urea, results in the production of urine hyperosmotic to plasma by providing the osmotic driving force for water reabsorption from the collecting duct. The overall process is termed **countercurrent multiplication**.

After the thick ascending limb, tubular fluid is hyperosmotic with respect to the surrounding interstitial fluid. In the presence of **ADH**, water channels (**aquaporins**) are inserted into the collecting duct and its water permeability increases. As a result, water diffuses out of the tubular lumen thus concentrating the urine. This process occurs throughout the length of the collecting duct and due to the increasing osmolality of the interstitial fluid with increasing medullary depth, the urine is concentrated further.

Urea is an important constituent of the **interstitial fluid** whose concentration increases with increasing depth into the medulla. The medullary collecting duct exhibits the highest permeability to urea. **ADH** increases the permeability of the terminal portion of the collecting duct to urea. As a result, urea diffuses into the interstitium thus increasing the urea concentration and thus increasing the reabsorption of H_2O. Low protein diets result in a reduced urea in the interstitial fluid. As a result, water reabsorption from the collecting duct is reduced and dilute urine is produced.

This mechanism is crucially dependent on the maintenance of the interstitium fluid osmolality gradients. Two structures achieve that: **Henle's loop** of the nephron **vasa recta** and the capillary network that supplies blood to the medulla. They are highly permeable to solute and H_2O and they remove excess water and solutes that are continuously added to the interstitium. In this way, they maintain the medullary interstitial gradient. However, this is **flow dependent**; if blood flow increases, then the gradient will ultimately disappear.

Answers

10. 1 – C, 2 – G, 3 – B, 4 – C, 5 – A, 6 – H

11. Regarding Na⁺

    a. It is the major cation in plasma
    b. Normal plasma concentration is 3.5–5.0 mM
    c. Its majority is complexed in bone
    d. It is the major determinant of the ICF
    e. It is the major determinant of the effective circulating volume

12. Regarding Na⁺ reabsorption by the nephron

    a. It is coupled to glucose in the first half of the proximal tubule
    b. It is coupled to H⁺ ion excretion in the second half of the proximal tubule
    c. It is reabsorbed via the paracellular pathway in the second half of the proximal tubule
    d. It is coupled to Cl⁻ ion reabsorption in the second half of the proximal tubule.
    e. It is reabsorbed coupled to lactate via an antiporter system in the first half of the proximal tubule

13. The diagram below represents a cell of the late distal tubule/collecting duct. Match the letters with the options next to it. Each option can be used once, more than once or not at all. Arrows indicate ion movements

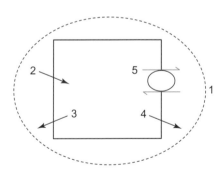

Options

    A. Intercalated cell   **B.** Principal cell
    C. Sodium ions   **D.** Potassium ions
    E. Na⁺/K⁺ ATPase   **F.** Chloride ions
    G. Hydrogen ions

ECF, extracellular fluid; ICF, intracellular fluid

EXPLANATION: SODIUM BALANCE AND THE KIDNEY

The body of an adult man contains approximately 3000 mmol of **Na$^+$**, 70 per cent of which is freely exchangeable and the remainder is complexed in bone. The majority of exchangeable Na$^+$ is **extracellular**; the normal plasma concentration is 135–145 mM. Na$^+$ is the major determinant of the **effective circulatory volume** (i.e. physiologically active ECF volume).

Approximately 67 per cent of filtered Na$^+$ is reabsorbed in the **proximal tubule**. In its first half, Na$^+$ reabsorption is coupled to that of HCO$_3^-$ and a number of organic molecules (e.g. glucose, lactate, amino acid) using **symporter** proteins. Na$^+$ is also reabsorbed here coupled to H$^+$ ion excretion via an antiporter protein. In the second half, Na$^+$ is reabsorbed coupled to Cl$^-$ by the operation of parallel Na$^+$/H$^+$ ions and Cl$^-$/base antiporters (base can be formate, oxalate, etc.). Na$^+$ is also reabsorbed here via the **paracellular** route coupled to Cl$^-$ movement generated by the high Cl$^-$ concentration in tubular fluid.

Henle's loop reabsorbs about 20 per cent of the remaining Na$^+$ (by the mechanism discussed before) and the distal tubule and collecting duct about 12 per cent. In the early part of the distal tubule, Na$^+$ is reabsorbed coupled to Cl$^-$ via a Na$^+$/Cl$^-$ symporter. The last segments of the distal tubule and the collecting duct are composed of two cell types, principal and intercalated cells. **Principal cells** reabsorb Na$^+$ and water and secrete K$^+$. Both processes depend on the activity of the **Na$^+$/K$^+$ ATPase** pump in the basolateral membrane to generate the electrochemical forces dictating these processes. The net result is that only 1 per cent of filtered Na$^+$ is lost in the urine.

Answers

11. T F F F T
12. T F T T F
13. 1 – B, 2 – C, 3 – D, 4 – D, 5 – E

14. Regarding the effective circulatory volume

    a. It is the same as the ECF volume
    b. It is determined by the amount of NaCl in ECF
    c. It is not measurable
    d. It determines renal Na$^+$ excretion
    e. Its decrease causes diuresis

15. Regarding the regulation of the effective circulating volume (ECV)

    a. It is controlled only by hormonal signals
    b. Low-pressure volume receptors are situated in the pulmonary vasculature
    c. High-pressure baroreceptors are situated in the kidneys' efferent arterioles
    d. Signals from volume sensors can modulate ADH secretion
    e. Signals from volume sensors modulate parasympathetic nerves in the kidneys

16. Regarding the regulation of the effective circulating volume

    a. Sympathetic nerves innervate the afferent arterioles
    b. Parasympathetic nerves innervate the efferent arterioles
    c. Renal sympathetic nerves cause renin secretion
    d. Renal sympathetic nerves decrease GFR when activated
    e. Sympathetic nerves in the kidneys are inhibited by an increase in ECV

ADH, anti-diuretic hormone; ECF, extracellular fluid; ECV, effective circulating volume; GFR, glomerular filtration rate

EXPLANATION: EFFECTIVE CIRCULATORY VOLUME – MONITORING AND REGULATION

The effective circulating volume (ECV) is not a measurable and distinct body fluid compartment; it is rather related to the adequacy of the tissue perfusion. It represents the 'fullness' and 'pressure' within the vascular tree. This volume is determined by the NaCl amount present and determines Na^+ excretion by the kidneys. An increase causes **natriuresis** and a decrease causes **antinatriuresis**.

Volume sensors can sense changes in ECV. The **low-pressure receptors** are found in the pulmonary vasculature and cardiac atria. The **high-pressure baroreceptors** are located in the aortic arch, the carotid sinus and the afferent arterioles of the kidneys. Activity of both types of sensors modulates both sympathetic outflow and ADH secretion. A decrease in ECV is sensed and increases **sympathetic** nerve activity and stimulated **ADH secretion**. Conversely, an increase in ECV has the opposite effect.

Sympathetic nerve fibres innervate the **afferent** and **efferent arterioles**. When activated (as above), they constrict the arterioles causing a reduction in **glomerular filtration rate (GFR)**; they also stimulate renin secretion by the kidney and they increase NaCl reabsorption by the proximal tubule and Henle's loop. These responses are mediated via the activation of alpha-adrenergic receptors. The net result is to reduce the excretion of NaCl, thus counteracting the change in the ECV.

Answers
14. F T T T F
15. F T F T F
16. T F T T T

17. Regarding the renin–angiotensin–aldosterone system

    a. Renin is released by the juxtaglomerular apparatus
    b. The efferent arteriole stimulates renin secretion when its perfusion pressure is reduced
    c. Renin causes vasoconstriction of the afferent arteriole
    d. Renin secretion is enhanced when NaCl delivery to the macula densa is increased
    e. Angiotensinogen is synthesized in the mesangium of the kidney

18. Regarding the renin–angiotensin–aldosterone system

    a. Angiotensin I stimulates the release of aldosterone
    b. Angiotensin II stimulates thirst
    c. Angiotensin I stimulates ADH secretion
    d. At high concentrations angiotensin II increases GFR
    e. Angiotensin III inhibits the release of aldosterone

19. Regarding aldosterone and atrial natriuretic peptide (ANP)

    a. Aldosterone stimulates the synthesis of Na^+/K^+ ATPase pumps
    b. Aldosterone is a protein synthesized in the adrenal cortex
    c. ANP inhibits aldosterone release by the adrenal gland
    d. ANP dilates the afferent arteriole of the kidney
    e. ANP counteracts the actions of aldosterone in the collecting duct

ACE, angiotensin converting enzyme; ADH, anti-diuretic hormone; ANP, atrial natriuretic peptide; ECV, extracellular volume; GFR, glomerular filtration rate; JGA, juxtaglomerular apparatus; PCT, proximal convoluted tubule

EXPLANATION: EFFECTIVE CIRCULATORY VOLUME REGULATION – RENIN–ANGIOTENSIN–ALDOSTERONE SYSTEM

The **renin–angiotensin–aldosterone** system is a means of regulating **GFR**. It is initiated by solute detectors in the **macula densa**, which stimulates the **juxtaglomerular apparatus (JGA)** in the wall of the afferent arteriole. Cells of the JGA secrete renin. Renin is an enzyme which converts angiotensinogen to angiotensin I, then **angiotensin converting enzyme (ACE)** mainly in the lung converts **angiotensin I** to **angiotensin II**.

The stimulus for this process is a **decrease** in the effective circulating volume. **Angiotensin II** stimulates **aldosterone** release, ADH secretion and thirst, arteriolar vasoconstriction (at low concentrations increases GFR) and enhancement of NaCl reabsorption by the proximal tubule. Its actions are terminated by plasma peptidases, which convert it to angiotensin III.

Aldosterone is a steroid hormone which is mainly synthesized and released by the cells of the zona glomerulosa of the **adrenal cortex**. Its release is triggered by angiotensin II and hyperkalaemia. It acts on distal tubules and collecting ducts and stimulates the synthesis of Na^+/K^+ ATPase pumps, insertion of Na^+-conductance channels into apical membranes and insertion of thiazide-sensitive NaCl channels in distal tubules.

ANP is a peptide hormone released by the atria. It is released in response to **atrial stretch** (i.e. increase in ECV). Its actions include: dilatation of the afferent arteriole; inhibition or renin, aldosterone and ADH release; and direct inhibition of NaCl reabsorption by the proximal convoluted tubule (PCT). The net result is a natriuresis.

Answers
17. T F F F F
18. F T F F F
19. T F T T F

20. The diagram below illustrates an integrated response to a decrease in the effective circulating volume. Match the letters to the options. Each option can be used once, more than once or not at all

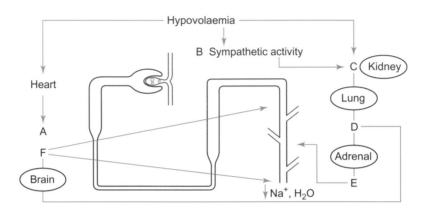

Options

A. Increased ANP production
B. Reduced ANP production
C. Increased
D. Decreased
E. Renin
F. Angiotensin I
G. Angiotensin II
H. Increased aldosterone
I. Decreased aldosterone
J. Increased ADH production
K. Reduced ADH production

ADH, anti-diuretic hormone; ANP, atrial natriuretic peptide; ECV, extracellular volume; GFR, glomerular filtration rate

EXPLANATION: REGULATION OF EXTRACELLULAR VOLUME – AN INTEGRATED VIEW

When the **ECV is decreased**, Na$^+$ and **H$_2$O** excretion by the kidneys is reduced. The entire nephron contributes to this response. The three general responses to a decrease in the ECV are:

1. The **GFR** and hence the filtered Na$^+$ load is reduced. This occurs due to the afferent and efferent arteriolar contraction effected by the increased sympathetic activity.

2. **Na$^+$ reabsorption** by the **proximal tubule** is stimulated as a result of the increased sympathetic activity and the direct action of angiotensin II.

3. **Na$^+$ reabsorption** by the **collecting** duct is enhanced. This is stimulated mainly by the action of aldosterone. Other hormones may also contribute here. ANP levels are reduced and ADH levels are elevated. ADH not only stimulates Na$^+$ reabsorption but also increases water reabsorption by the collecting duct. As a result, the urine can be rendered virtually Na$^+$-free. The net effect is a restoration of the ECV.

The above example applies to **hypovolaemia**. The converse is true for hypervolaemia. Of course, in both cases, physiological mechanisms can only compensate if the disturbance is within their functional limits (i.e. excessive, continuous bleeding is beyond these limits).

Answers

20. 1 – B, 2 – C, 3 – E, 4 – G, 5 – H, 6 – J

21. Regarding potassium homeostasis

a. Most K$^+$ lies within cells
b. Extracellular [K$^+$] is 4–5 mM
c. The gastrointestinal tract is the major route of K$^+$ excretion from the body
d. Adrenaline does not affect K$^+$ excretion by the kidneys
e. Insulin stimulates K$^+$ uptake into cells

22. Regarding potassium homeostasis

a. Aldosterone promotes K$^+$ uptake into cells
b. Stimulation of beta$_2$-adrenoceptors decreases plasma [K$^+$]
c. High plasma osmolality increases extracellular [K$^+$]
d. Excessive exercise can cause a decrease in plasma [K$^+$]
e. A rise in ADH increases uptake of K$^+$ into cells

23. Regarding potassium and acid–base balance:

a. Metabolic acidosis decreases plasma [K$^+$]
b. Respiratory acidosis decreases plasma [K$^+$]
c. Metabolic alkalosis decreases plasma [K$^+$]
d. Accumulation of organic acids causes a lower rise in plasma [K$^+$] than inorganic acids
e. Lactic acid accumulation in plasma causes an increase in plasma [K$^+$]

ADH, anti-diuretic hormone; ECF, extracellular fluid

EXPLANATION: POTASSIUM HOMEOSTASIS AND NON-RENAL CONTROL MECHANISMS

K^+ is the most abundant **intracellular** cation. Its average concentration within cells is **135–145 mM** and its average extracellular concentration is **4–5 mM**. This large concentration difference is maintained by the operation of the **Na^+/K^+ ATPase** pumps. This gradient is important for the excitability of nerve and muscle cells as well as for the contractility of cardiac, skeletal and smooth muscle cells. K^+ balance depends on the regulation of its ECF distribution and its renal excretion.

Catecholamines (e.g. adrenaline) stimulate beta$_2$-receptors and cause increased uptake of K^+ into cells. **Insulin** and **aldosterone** also exert similar effects. These hormones are the major physiological factors keeping plasma $[K^+]$ constant.

In contrast, plasma **osmolality** perturbs plasma $[K^+]$. High osmolality shifts water extracellularly and K^+ flows out of cells down a now-steeper concentration gradient. Cell lysis (due to trauma or tumours) releases K^+ into the ECF. Exercise also causes an increase in plasma K^+ due to the increased leakage of K^+ during the recovery phase of the action potential.

Finally, **acid–base disorders** alter plasma $[K^+]$. **Metabolic acidosis** causes an increase in plasma $[K^+]$ and metabolic alkalosis, a decrease. **Respiratory acid–base disorders** have little effect on plasma $[K^+]$. The acidosis causes H^+ ions to move into cells and K^+ to move out to maintain the electrical charge. This effect is greatest with the addition of inorganic acids. Organic acids do not exert such a profound effect probably due to simultaneous shifting of organic anions into cells.

Answers

21. T T F T T
22. T T T F F
23. F F T T T

24. Regarding the renal handling of potassium

a. Seventy per cent of filtered K^+ is absorbed in the proximal tubule
b. The loop of Henle (thick ascending limb) can secrete K^+ into tubular fluid
c. K^+ is secreted into tubular fluid by a pump at the apical surface of the collecting duct
d. K^+ is secreted into tubular fluid by the principal cells of the collecting duct
e. High plasma $[K^+]$ increases the permeability of the basolateral membrane of the collecting duct cells to K^+

25. Regarding hormones and the renal handling of potassium

a. ADH increases K^+ secretion by the distal tubule
b. ADH increases the urinary excretion of K^+
c. Aldosterone increases secretion of K^+ by increasing Na^+–K^+ ATPase numbers in collecting duct intercalated cells
d. Aldosterone secretion is inhibited by a high plasma $[K^+]$
e. ADH increases the electrochemical driving force for K^+ exit from collecting duct cells

26. Regarding acid–base balance and the renal handling of potassium

a. Alkalosis increases K^+ excretion
b. Acidosis increases K^+ excretion
c. The effect of metabolic acidosis on K^+ excretion is time independent
d. Acidosis increases the permeability of the apical membrane of the distal tubule cells to K^+
e. Alkalosis increases the permeability of the apical membrane of the distal tubule cells to K^+

ADH, anti-diuretic hormone

EXPLANATION: POTASSIUM HOMEOSTASIS AND THE KIDNEY

The kidneys play the major role in **maintaining K⁺ balance**. The primary event in determining urinary K⁺ excretion is K⁺ secretion from the blood into the tubular fluid by the **principal cells** of the distal tubule and collecting duct system.

The **renal handling** of K⁺ is depicted below.

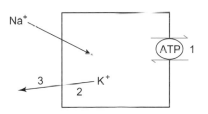

Factors determining K⁺ secretion:
1. Na^+/K^+ATPase activity
2. Electrochemical potential gradient
3. K⁺ permeability

Many regulators affect the renal handling of K⁺. High **plasma [K⁺]** increases K⁺ secretion by increasing all the above factors. **Aldosterone** secretion is increased by hyperkalaemia and stimulates K⁺ secretion by increasing all the above factors. The flow of tubular fluid can also affect K⁺ secretion. A rise in the flow stimulates K⁺ secretion because there is increased wash-out of secreted K⁺. **ADH** has no effect in the urinary excretion of K⁺. ADH levels increase the electrochemical potential gradient of K⁺ across the apical membrane (factor 2 above), but reduce tubular fluid flow thus leading to a constant urinary K⁺ excretion.

Finally, **acid–base balance** affects urinary K⁺ excretion. An acute acidosis decreases K⁺ secretion by inhibiting factors 1 and 3. However, in chronic acidosis, K⁺ secretion is increased; this happens because it causes a rise in tubular fluid flow and plasma [K⁺] and increased aldosterone production.

Answers
24. T F F T F
25. F F F F T
26. T F T F T

27. Regarding sodium balance disturbances

   a. Thiazide diuretics can cause hyponatraemia
   b. Hypernatraemia causes thirst
   c. Cirrhosis can cause hyponatraemia
   d. Lung tumours can cause hyponatraemia
   e. Conn's syndrome can cause hyponatraemia

28. Regarding potassium balance disturbances

   a. Intestinal fistulae can cause hyperkalaemia
   b. Burns can cause hypokalaemia
   c. Hypokalaemia is corrected by administering a fast bolus dose of K^+
   d. Spironolactone can cause hypokalaemia
   e. Alkalosis can cause hypokalaemia

29. Below there is a list of electrocardiographic changes. Indicate which of them would be found in a patient with hypokalaemia

   a. Small T waves
   b. Prominent U waves
   c. Shortened PR interval
   d. Depressed ST segment
   e. Prolonged PR interval
   f. Peaked T waves
   g. Absent P waves

ADH, anti-diuretic hormone; ACE, angiotensin converting enzyme

EXPLANATION: SODIUM AND POTASSIUM DISTURBANCES – CAUSES AND CLINICAL EFFECTS

Normal plasma [Na⁺] is 135–145 mM. If [Na⁺] is greater than 145 mM then **hypernatraemia** exists, whereas below 135 mM **hyponatraemia** exists. The former can cause thirst, confusion, fits and even coma. It is usually caused by water loss in excess of Na⁺ loss. Conditions that can cause hypernatraemia include **diarrhoea** and vomiting, **diabetes insipidus** and **hyperaldosteronism** (e.g. Conn's syndrome). Hyponatraemia can also cause fits but it usually produces **confusion, nausea, muscle weakness, hypotension** and even **cardiac failure**. Causes include **diuretics** especially thiazides, iatrogenic excess saline administration, cirrhosis and renal failure. Inappropriate **ADH** secretion (after head injury or malignant tumours) can also cause hyponatraemia.

Normal plasma [K⁺] is 3.5–5 mM. If it is greater that 5 mM then hyperkalaemia is present whereas if it is below 3.5 mM, hypokalaemia exists. The diagrams below indicate the ECG changes in hypokalaemia and hyperkalaemia.

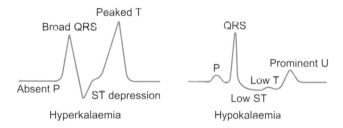

Causes of **hyperkalaemia** include **K⁺-sparing** diuretics (spironolactone, amiloride), metabolic acidosis, burns and **ACE inhibitors**. Causes of **hypokalaemia** include alkalosis, vomiting and diarrhoea, intestinal fistulae and Conn's syndrome. Both types of K⁺ disturbance can be deadly since they cause **cardiac arrhythmias**. Hypokalaemia **must never** be corrected using a fast 'stat' bolus dose and hyperkalaemia can be corrected temporarily with insulin and dextrose.

Answers

27. T T T T F
28. F F F F T
29. T T T T F F F

30. Regarding plasma pH

a. The normal range is 7.40–7.45
b. The normal range for HCO_3^- is 24–26 mM
c. A pH value of below 7.1 is an alkalosis
d. pH is the positive logarithm of the H^+ concentration
e. It is principally maintained in the normal range by buffers

31. Regarding the buffering of hydrogen ions

a. A buffer is a weak acid
b. PO_4^{3-} is an important buffer in the ECF
c. A buffer prevents changes in plasma pH
d. The most important buffer system in blood is the HCO_3^-/CO_2 system
e. Buffers are ineffective when the pH is close to their pK

32. Regarding the buffering of hydrogen ions

a. Respiratory rate is a major determinant of arterial CO_2 concentration
b. NH_3 is an important buffer in the kidneys
c. The enzyme carbonic decarboxylase catalyses the reaction: $H_2CO_3 = H^+ + HCO_3^-$
d. Buffers combine irreversibly with H^+ ions
e. The Henderson–Hasselbalch equation allows the calculation of pH for a given concentration of CO_2 and HCO_3^-

ECF, extracellular fluid

EXPLANATION: pH AND HYDROGEN IONS

The **pH** is the negative logarithm of the H^+ ion concentration. Plasma pH is normally 7.4 and is normally maintained within the range **7.35 –7.45**. **Acidosis** is plasma pH below 7.35 whereas **alkalosis** is plasma pH above 7.45. If plasma pH goes below 7.1 or above 7.7, this may be fatal. The body has three mechanisms for regulating pH: **buffers**, the **lungs** and the **kidneys**.

A **buffer** is a weak acid or base that can combine reversibly with H^+ ions. It has two characteristics that determine its effectiveness: its **concentration** and its **pK.** This is the negative logarithm of its dissociation constant and also the pH at which half of it is dissociated or undissociated. Buffers are generally only effective when the pH is within one unit of the pK. The **main buffers** are proteins, NH_3 (kidney), PO_4^{3-} (kidney), CO_2, urate and citrate. A buffer cannot prevent a pH change when an acid or alkali is added; it can only make the change in pH smaller than it would have been without the buffer.

The most important buffers are the **HCO_3^-/CO_2 system**:

$$CO_2 + H_2O = H_2CO_3 = H^+ + HCO_3^-$$

The first part is catalysed by **carbonic anhydrase**. The second part is fast. If both reactions are in equilibrium, the **Henderson–Hasselbalch** equation applies:

$$pH = 6.1 + \log_{10} [HCO_3^-] / [\alpha P_{CO_2}]$$
$$\alpha = \text{a constant equal to } 0.03$$
$$\alpha \times P_{CO_2} = [H_2CO_3^-] \text{ mM}$$
$$\text{where } P_{CO_2} = 40 \text{ mm Hg}$$
$$H_2CO_3^- = 1.2 \text{ mM}$$

CO_2 is the major factor determining ventilation rate. An increase in P_{CO_2} results in an increase in ventilation and increased loss of CO_2 from the body. This effect helps to buffer changes in blood pH brought about by addition of acid and alkali.

Answers
30. F T F F F
31. T F F T F
32. T T F F T

33. Indicate the outcome of the following metabolic reactions using the options below. Each option can be used once, more than once or not at all

Options

A. Volatile acid
B. Titratable acid
C. Non-titratable acid
D. Weak acid
E. Strong acid
F. Weak base
G. Strong base

1. Carbohydrate oxidative metabolism
2. Glucose anaerobic metabolism
3. Cysteine oxidation
4. Urate anaerobic metabolism
5. Lysine oxidation

EXPLANATION: BIOLOGICAL ACIDS AND HYDROGEN ION BALANCE

Oxidative metabolism of carbohydrates and fats produces CO_2, 12–20 moles per day, and is excreted by the lungs. Hydration of CO_2 forms carbonic acid H_2CO_3, this partially dissociates to H^+ and HCO_3^- but this process is reversed in the lungs and there is no permanent addition of acid to the body fluids. Acid that can be lost via the lungs (because it is CO_2) is called **volatile acid** (H_2CO_3).

Other metabolic processes lead to the production of **weak acids** (lactate from anaerobic metabolism of glucose, citrate, urate) or **strong acids** (H_2SO_4 from cysteine or HCl from lysine). Oxidation of a neutral amino acid (glutamine) leads to production of NH_4^+ and HCO_3^- ions. These cannot be excreted in the lungs but they can be **excreted** in the **kidneys**. Acid excreted in the urine is called **fixed** acid; the acid that can be measured by titration to pH 7 with NaOH is called **titratable** acid. Titratable acid excludes the H^+ ions present as NH_4^+ ions.

Answers

33. 1 – A, 2 – D, 3 – E, 4 – D, 5 – G

34. Regarding the excretion of acid into urine

a. 70–100 mmoles H^+ are excreted daily in the urine in a healthy adult
b. The pH of urine is usually below 7.0
c. The minimum pH of urine is 4.6
d. Urinary NH_3 is the principal urinary buffer
e. Net acid excretion equals the volatile and non-volatile acid production

35. Regarding the reabsorption of HCO_3^-

a. All the filtered HCO_3^- is reabsorbed in a healthy individual
b. The luminal surface of renal tubular cells is permeable to CO_2
c. Most HCO_3^- is absorbed by the loop of Henle
d. It is absorbed by the collecting duct
e. The renal threshold for its reabsorption depends on the $P{CO_2}$

36. Regarding the regulation of acid secretion and HCO_3^- reabsorption

a. Acclimatization to altitude decreases the renal threshold for HCO_3^- reabsorption
b. Aldosterone increases acid secretion by the distal convoluted tubule
c. Acetazolamide decreases the reabsorption of HCO_3^-
d. Acetazolamide decreases the secretion of H^+ ions
e. Glutaminase is essential for the excretion of H^+ ions

EXPLANATION: RENAL HANDLING OF HYDROGEN ION BALANCE – BASIC CONCEPTS

To maintain **acid–base balance**, the kidneys must excrete an amount of acid equal to the non-volatile acid production. In addition, they must prevent the loss of HCO_3^- in the urine.

Both the **reabsorption** of the filtered load of HCO_3^- and the **excretion** of acid are accomplished through the process of H^+ secretion by the nephrons. **Carbonic anhydrase** is essential for both processes so its inhibition by acetazolamide inhibits them both. In a single day, the nephrons secrete about 400 mmoles of H^+ ions. Most of these ions are not excreted in the urine but they serve to reclaim the filtered load of HCO_3^-. Only 70 mmoles are excreted per day. As a result, the urine is normally acidic (i.e. pH <7.0).

Glomerular filtration delivers 4320 mmoles of HCO_3^- to the proximal tubule. Approximately 85 per cent of this HCO_3^- **is reabsorbed** by this segment. The luminal surface of renal tubular cells is impermeable to HCO_3^- and therefore direct reabsorption cannot occur. An additional 10 per cent is absorbed by **Henle's loop**, and the **distal tubule** and **collecting duct** absorb the remaining 5 per cent.

HCO_3^- is normally completely reabsorbed up to a renal threshold. This is higher than the normal plasma HCO_3^- and corresponds to alkalosis. This threshold varies with the Pco_2 of blood. At high altitude, low atmospheric Po_2 **stimulates respiration** which leads to a **fall in Pco_2**. This fall leads to a reduction in HCO_3^- excretion in the urine. This is renal compensation for **respiratory alkalosis**.

The **minimum urinary pH** that can be generated is 4.6. Given a normal urine volume, free H^+ excretion can account for less than 0.1 per cent of the total amount that has to be excreted. The principal urinary buffer is PO_4^{3-} accompanied by NH_3 (it is produced from glutamine via the action of glutaminase).

Answers
34. T T T F F
35. T T F T T
36. T F T T T

37. The diagram below represents a proximal tubule cell of a nephron. Match the labelled structures with the options below. Each option can be used once, more than once or not at all. The arrows represent molecular movement

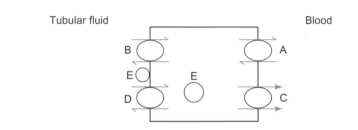

Options

A. Na^+/K^+ ATPase
B. Na^+/H^+ ion antiporter
C. Carbonic anhydrase
D. HCO_3^-
E. CO_2
F. $HCO_3^- - Cl^-$ antiporter
G. Na^+/HCO_3^- symporter

EXPLANATION: RENAL HANDLING OF BICARBONATE IONS

The **glomerular filtrate** contains the same concentration of HCO_3^- ions as plasma. In health, at normal plasma HCO_3^- concentrations, virtually all the filtered HCO_3^- is reabsorbed.

The **luminal surface** of renal tubular cells is impermeable to HCO_3^- and therefore direct reabsorption cannot occur. Within the renal tubular cells, carbonic acid, H_2CO_3 is formed from CO_2 and water via the action of the enzyme **carbonic anhydrase**. The H_2CO_3 then dissociates to give H^+ and HCO_3^- **ions**. The formation of HCO_3^- and H^+ ions is promoted by their continuous removal and by the presence of carbonic anhydrase. HCO_3^- crosses the basal border of the cells into the interstitial fluid. The H^+ **ions** are secreted across the luminal membrane in exchange for Na^+ ions. HCO_3^- is co-transported across the basolateral membrane with Na^+.

In most **tubular fluid**, H^+ ions combine with HCO_3^- to form H_2CO_3, most of which dissociates into CO_2 and water. Some of the CO_2 diffuses back into the renal tubular cells while the remainder is excreted in the urine. This whole process effectively results in the **reabsorption** of filtered HCO_3^-.

Answers
37. 1 – A, 2 – B, 3 – D, 4 – F, 5 – C.

38. The following diagram represents a proximal tubule cell of a nephron. Match the labelled structures with the options below. Each option can be used once, more than once or not at all. Arrows represent molecular movement

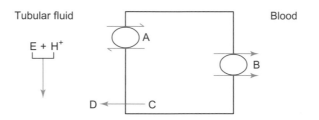

Tubular fluid   Blood

E + H⁺

Options

A. Na^+/H^+ antiporter
B. Na^+/HCO_3^- symporter
C. K^+/HCO_3^- symporter
D. NH_3
E. NH_4^+
F. HPO_4^{2-}
G. $H_2PO_4^-$

EXPLANATION: RENAL HANDLING OF HYDROGEN IONS

H^+ and HCO_3^- ions are generated in renal tubular cells from CO_2 and water. The H^+ ions are excreted in the urine and are buffered by PO_4^{3-} and NH_3.

The principal **urinary buffer** is PO_4^{3-}. This is present in the glomerular filtrate, approximately 80 per cent being in the form of the divalent anion, HPO_4^{2-}. This combines with H^+ ions and is converted to $H_2PO_4^-$. About 30–40 mmoles of H^+ ions are normally excreted in this way every 24 hours.

NH_3, produced by the deamination of glutamine in renal tubular cells, is also an important urinary buffer. The enzyme that catalyses this reaction, **glutaminase**, is induced in states of chronic acidosis, allowing increased NH_3 production and, hence, increased H^+ ion excretion via NH_4^+ ions. NH_3 can readily diffuse across cell membranes but NH_4^+ ions, formed when NH_3 buffers H^+ ions, cannot. Passive reabsorption of NH_4^+ ions is therefore prevented.

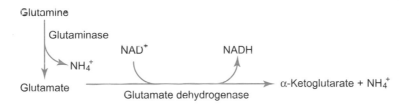

Answers

38. 1 – A, 2 – B, 3 – D, 4 – E, 5 – F

39. Regarding metabolic acidosis

a. It is characterized by a low plasma HCO_3^- and a low plasma pH
b. It is characterized by a high plasma HCO_3^- and a low plasma pH
c. It can be caused by salicylate overdose
d. It can be caused by diarrhoea
e. P_{CO_2} is reduced

40. Regarding respiratory acidosis

a. It is characterized by a reduced P_{O_2} and reduced plasma pH
b. Emphysema can cause it
c. NH_4^+ excretion by the kidneys is stimulated
d. Renal compensation is immediate
e. The anion gap is increased

41. Regarding acidosis

a. In renal tubular acidosis type 1, there is impaired HCO_3^- reabsorption from the proximal convoluted tubule
b. Diabetic ketoacidosis increases the anion gap
c. The reduction in P_{O_2} stimulates the respiratory centres in respiratory acidosis
d. Acidosis can cause paraesthesiae
e. Congestive cardiac failure can cause respiratory acidosis

COPD, chronic obstructive pulmonary disorder; ECF, extracellular fluid; ICF, intracellular fluid

EXPLANATION: ACIDOSIS – CAUSES AND COMPENSATORY MECHANISMS

An **acidosis** exists when plasma pH is below 7.35. This causes a variety of symptoms. The commonest are **hyperventilation**, **headaches** and **confusion**. To diagnose it, **H⁺ concentration** in **arterial blood**, anti-coagulated with heparin, is measured.

Acidosis can be categorized into **metabolic** and **respiratory**. **Metabolic acidosis** is characterized by a low plasma HCO_3^- concentration (<22 mM) and low plasma pH. Common causes are **diabetes (ketoacidosis)**, lactic acidosis, acid poisoning, diarrhoea and **renal tubular acidosis**. The latter is divided into two types: type 1 is due to an inability to excrete H⁺ ions whereas type 2 is due to impaired HCO_3^- reabsorption. The rise in H⁺ ions is initially buffered in both the ICF and ECF. The fall in pH will stimulate the respiratory centres and the ventilatory rate will increase (respiratory compensation). This reduces the P_{CO_2}, which helps minimize the fall in pH.

Respiratory acidosis is characterized by an elevated plasma P_{CO_2} (>45 mmHg) and reduced plasma pH. It can be due to an **airway obstruction** (chronic obstructive pulmonary disorder (COPD), aspiration, neuromuscular disease (poliomyelitis, curare, motor neuron disease), pulmonary disease (pulmonary fibrosis) and respiratory centre depression (anaesthetics, tumours). In contrast to the **metabolic disorders**, buffering during respiratory acidosis occurs almost entirely in the intracellular compartment (acute phase). In this type of acidosis, kidneys are stimulated to increase HCO_3^- reabsorption and NH_4^+ excretion (renal compensation). However, the renal compensatory response takes several days and occurs in the chronic phase of the disorder.

The **anion gap** is the difference between the sums of the concentrations of the principal cations (Na⁺ and K⁺) and the principal anions (Cl⁻ and HCO_3^-):

$$\text{Anion gap} = ([Na^+] + [K^+]) - ([Cl^-] + [HCO_3^-])$$

In health, the anion gap has a value of 14–18 mM and mainly represents the unmeasured net negative charge on plasma proteins. In an acidosis in which anions other than Cl⁻ are increased, the anion gap is increased. In contrast, in an acidosis due to loss of HCO_3^-, the plasma Cl⁻ concentration in increased and the anion gap is normal.

Answers
39. T T T T T
40. F T T F F
41. F T F T T

42. Match the diagnoses with the clinical scenarios below. Each diagnosis can be used once, more than once or not at all. (Normal values: pH $= 7.40$, $[HCO_3^-] = 24$ mM, $P_{CO_2} = 40$ mmHg)

Options

A. Metabolic acidosis with respiratory compensation
B. Metabolic acidosis with renal compensation
C. Metabolic alkalosis with respiratory compensation
D. Metabolic alkalosis with renal compensation
E. Respiratory acidosis with renal compensation (chronic respiratory acidosis)
F. Respiratory acidosis without renal compensation (acute respiratory acidosis)
G. Metabolic acidosis and respiratory acidosis

1. An individual with cardiopulmonary arrest: pH $= 7.23$, $[HCO_3^-] = 11$mM, $P_{CO_2} = 58$ mmHg
2. An individual with diabetes mellitus who forgets to take insulin: pH $= 7.29$, $[HCO_3^-] = 11$ mM, $P_{CO_2} = 24$ mmHg
3. An individual with an asthma attack: pH $= 7.28$, $[HCO_3^-] = 25$ mM, $P_{CO_2} = 55$ mmHg
4. An individual with a gastric ulcer who ingests large quantities of antacids: pH $= 7.49$, $[HCO_3^-] = 32$mM, $P_{CO_2} = 43$ mmHg
5. An individual with persistent diarrhoea: pH $= 7.34$, $[HCO_3^-] = 17$ mM, $P_{CO_2} = 32$ mmHg.

EXPLANATION: BIOCHEMICAL CLASSIFICATION OF ACID–BASE DISORDERS

Analysis of a clinical **acid–base** disorder is directed at identification of the underlying disorder so that appropriate therapy can be initiated. Usually, the patient's medical history produces valuable clues about the nature and origin of an acid–base disorder. However, an analysis of an **arterial blood** sample (**'blood gases'**) is frequently required.

Most **acid–base** disorders can be explained using a simple approach. Firstly, the **plasma pH** should be studied for an acidosis or an alkalosis. The defence mechanisms of the body cannot correct an acid–base disorder by themselves, they just compensate for it. So even if they are completely operative, the pH will still indicate the origin of the initial disorder.

Then we have to determine if the disorder is **metabolic or respiratory**. For this, the **HCO_3^-** and **$P\text{co}_2$** must be examined. If the $P\text{co}_2$ is abnormal and in keeping with the pH (i.e. if there is an acidosis, the $P\text{co}_2$ is raised), the problem is respiratory. If the HCO_3^- is abnormal and in keeping with the pH (i.e. if there is an alkalosis, the HCO_3^- is raised), the problem is metabolic.

Finally, the compensatory response can be analysed. Metabolic disorders result in **compensatory changes** in ventilation and hence $P\text{co}_2$. Respiratory disorders elicit compensatory changes in the renal acid excretion and thus in plasma HCO_3^-. If the compensatory response is not appropriate, a mixed acid–base disorder should be suspected. A mixed disorder simply reflects the presence of two or more underlying causes for the disturbances.

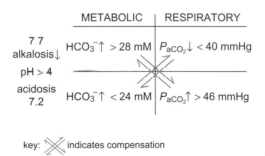

	METABOLIC	RESPIRATORY
7.7 alkalosis↓	$HCO_3^-\uparrow\ >28$ mM	$P_{aCO_2}\downarrow\ <40$ mmHg
pH > 4		
acidosis 7.2	$HCO_3^-\uparrow\ <24$ mM	$P_{aCO_2}\uparrow\ >46$ mmHg

key: ✕ indicates compensation

---

43. Calcium

    a. Is essential for effective blood coagulation
    b. Circulates in plasma predominantly bound to proteins
    c. Concentration in plasma is 4 mM
    d. Is essential for neurotransmitter uptake from synaptic clefts
    e. Is essential for neurotransmitter release

44. Regarding calcium homeostasis

    a. The majority of ingested Ca^{2+} is lost in the faeces
    b. Absorption of ingested Ca^{2+} is increased by calcitonin
    c. Absorption of ingested Ca^{2+} occurs by an active process
    d. Filtered Ca^{2+} can be reabsorbed by the loop of Henle
    e. Ca^{2+} reabsorption by the distal tubule occurs by a paracellular pathway

45. Regarding calcium homeostasis

    a. Ca^{2+} bound to citrate does not get filtered through the glomeruli
    b. Parathyroid hormone (PTH) increases Ca^{2+} reabsorption by the kidneys
    c. Ca^{2+} reabsorbed by the proximal tubule diffuses into the blood down its electrochemical gradient
    d. Ca^{2+} is extruded across the basal membrane of distal tubule cells by a Ca^{2+}/ATPase
    e. Ca^{2+} reabsorption by the proximal tubule occurs via a transcellular pathway

1,25$[OH]_2D_3$, 1,25-dihydroxyvitamin D_3; ECF, extracellular fluid; ICF, intracellular fluid; PTH, parathyroid hormone

EXPLANATION: CALCIUM BALANCE

Ca²⁺ plays a major role in bone formation, cell division, blood coagulation and signal transduction in cells. Ninety-nine per cent of Ca^{2+} is in bone and 1 per cent in the ICF. Total plasma Ca^{2+} concentration is about 2.5 mM. Fifty per cent of this is ionized, 45 per cent is bound to proteins (albumin) and 5 per cent is bound to anions (citrate).

Ca^{2+} balance is achieved by regulating its absorption from the **gastrointestinal** tract, its distribution between the ICF and the ECF and its excretion by the kidneys. Ca^{2+} absorption by the gut occurs by an active, carrier-mediated transport system and is increased by **1,25-dihydroxyvitamin D₃ (1,25[OH]₂D₃).**

The **renal handling** of Ca^{2+} is shown below.

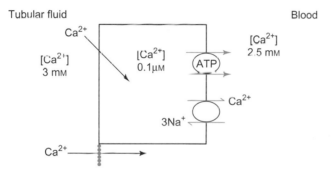

Ionized and anion-complexed Ca^{2+} is freely filtered at the glomeruli. Ca^{2+} reabsorption by the **proximal tubule** and the loop of Henle (thick ascending limb) is via the transcellular and paracellular pathways. Ca^{2+} in the distal tubule and collecting duct is reabsorbed via the transcellular pathway only. **PTH** dramatically stimulates Ca^{2+} absorption by Henle's loop and the distal tubule.

Answers
43. T F F F T
44. T F T T F
45. F T F T T

46. Regarding calcium balance disorders

    a. Hypercalcaemia can be caused by malignant tumours
    b. Hypocalcaemia can cause Chvostek's sign
    c. Hypercalcaemia predisposes to renal calculi
    d. Hypercalcaemia can be caused by renal failure
    e. Inadequate exposure to sunlight can cause hypocalcaemia

47. Regarding calcium balance disorders

    a. Hypercalcaemia can cause tetany
    b. Hypercalcaemia can cause Trousseau's sign
    c. Hypokalaemia can be caused by pancreatitis
    d. Hypercalcaemia causes a short QT interval on the electrocardiogram (ECG)
    e. Hypercalcaemia can be caused by hyperparathyroidism

48. Regarding calcium balance disorders

    a. Hypocalcaemia can cause carpopedal spasm
    b. Hypercalcaemia can cause perioral paraesthesiae
    c. Hypocalcaemia causes a short QT interval on ECG
    d. Hypocalcaemia can be caused by Mg^{2+} deficiency
    e. Hypercalcaemia can cause cardiac arrest

ECG, electrocardiogram, PTH, parathyroid hormone

EXPLANATION: CALCIUM BALANCE DISTURBANCES – CAUSES AND CLINICAL EFFECTS

Disorders of Ca^{2+} homeostasis are categorized into **hypocalcaemias** and **hypercalcaemias.**

Hypocalcaemia can be an artefact of hypoalbuminaemia (since Ca^{2+} is bound mainly to albumin in plasma). It can cause tetany, depression, perioral paraesthesiae, carpopedal spasm (wrist flexion and fingers drawn together) especially if the brachial artery is occluded with a blood pressure cuff (**Trousseau's sign**) and neuromuscular excitability (e.g. tapping over parotid gland causes facial muscles to twitch (**Chvostek's sign**). In the ECG there is widening of the QT interval. Hypocalcaemia can be due to **low vitamin D** (inadequate diet or sunlight exposure), parathyroid surgery, Mg^{2+} deficiency and pancreatitis.

Hypercalcaemia can cause abdominal pain, vomiting, depression, tiredness, **renal stones**, anorexia and weight loss. The ECG shows shortening of the QT interval and patients may develop **cardiac arrest**. Most common causes include **malignancy** (myeloma, bone metastases) and **primary hyperparathyroidism**. Other causes include sarcoidosis, vitamin D intoxication and thyrotoxicosis. The best discriminating features between bone metastases and **hyperparathyroidism** are low albumin, low Cl⁻ and alkalosis (all suggesting metastases). Raised plasma **PTH** strongly supports hyperparathyroidism.

Answers

46. T T T F T
47. F F T T T
48. T F F T T

49. Regarding phosphate balance

a. Most PO_4^{3-} filtered at the glomerulus is reabsorbed by the thick ascending limb of Henle's loop

b. PO_4^{3-} diffuses into proximal tubule cells down its electrochemical gradient

c. PTH stimulates PO_4^{3-} reabsorption by the proximal tubule

d. $1,25[OH]_2D_3$ stimulates PO_4^{3-} release from bone

e. PO_4^{3-} is reabsorbed by the distal tubule via a transcellular pathway

50. Regarding phosphate balance

a. Glucocorticoids inhibit PO_4^{3-} reabsorption by the proximal tubule

b. Acidosis increases urinary PO_4^{3-} excretion

c. Hyperphosphataemia is caused by renal failure

d. Hypophosphataemia can be caused by vitamin D deficiency

e. Renal failure increases PO_4^{3-} excretion

51. Regarding magnesium

a. It is an important enzyme cofactor

b. Most filtered Mg^{2+} is reabsorbed by the proximal tubule

c. Hypercalcaemia increases urinary Mg^{2+} excretion

d. Acidosis increases urinary Mg^{2+} excretion

e. PTH increases Mg^{2+} excretion

ATP, adenosine triphosphate; $1,25[OH]_2D_3$, 1,25-dihydroxyvitamin D_3; DNA, deoxyribose nucleic acid; ECF, extracellular fluid; PTH, parathyroid hormone; RNA, ribose nucleic acid

EXPLANATION: RENAL HANDLING OF MAGNESIUM AND PHOSPHATE

PO_4^{3-} is an important component of DNA, RNA, ATP and bone. It is also important for **acid–base balance** since it acts as an important buffer for H^+ ions in the kidneys. The plasma PO_4^{3-} concentration is 1.3 mM. Most of it is ionized and freely filtered at the glomerulus. The **renal handling** is shown below.

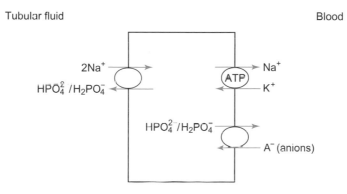

The **proximal tubule** reabsorbs most of the PO_4^{3-} via a transcellular pathway. The distal tubule reabsorbs about 10 per cent via unknown mechanisms. The **loop of Henle** and the collecting duct reabsorb tiny amounts. Many factors affect PO_4^{3-} balance. PTH increases PO_4^{3-} excretion. The same occurs with ECF expansion, glucocorticoids, dietary PO_4^{3-} loading and acidosis.

Mg^{2+} is an important **cofactor** for many enzymes. It is also important for bone formation. The plasma Mg^{2+} concentration is about 1 mM and most of it is ionized. The **kidneys** are vital in Mg^{2+} homeostasis and most of the filtered Mg^{2+} is reabsorbed by the thick ascending limb of Henle's loop via an uncharacterized mechanism. Many factors influence renal Mg^{2+} excretion. Hypercalcaemia, hypermagnesaemia, ECF expansion, acidosis and a decrease in plasma PTH concentration increase it.

Answers

49. F F F T F
50. T T T T T
51. T F T T F

INDEX